MISSION BETRAYED

How the VA Really Fails America's Vets

MISSION BETRAYED

How the VA Really Fails America's Vets

By

MICHAEL J. MANN, MD

PO Box 22487
San Francisco, CA 94122

ISBN-13: 978-0-692-77848-7
LCCN: 2016953875

Distributed by Itasca Books

Printed in the United States of America

This book is dedicated to my father, a veteran of the United States Army, without whom this book might never have been written, nor seen the light of day.

PREFACE

Way Beyond Waiting Lists

T he Veterans Health Administration is home to the United States's largest integrated healthcare system. It consists of 168 medical centers, and a total of more than 1,700 sites of care, including community-based outpatient clinics, community living centers, and vet centers. It has an annual budget of roughly $59 billion, employs over 25,000 doctors, and serves 9 million veterans each year.[1]

It's a system rooted in deep, increasingly malignant trouble.

By the summer of 2014, a constant trickle of news about the VA wait list scandal had grown into a flood of frightening daily disclosures. It had taken years for a single whistleblowing doctor's devastating revelations to be heard by a reluctant Congress. Delays in care were so expected that they alone could not get anyone's attention. And so the focus shifted to the resulting deaths. That delays were severe enough to result in veteran deaths certainly seemed unacceptable; but that VA administrators had orchestrated an intricate, nationwide program of deceit and had transformed those ugly statistics into a fabricated justification for their own professional and financial benefit was nothing less than horrifying.

But what if that was not the whole story? Numerous investigations, both internal and external—some instigated by the burgeoning waitlist

---

[1] "About VHA," http://www.va.gov/health/aboutVHA.asp; "Providing healthcare for veterans," http://www.va.gov/health/; "Become a VA physician," http://www.vacareers.va.gov/assets/common/print/Physician_Brochure.pdf; accessed August 25, 2016.

scandal, some that had been initiated even before it hit the front pages—began to hint at much more serious problems. A White House deputy chief of staff, Rob Nabors, was assigned to oversee a nationwide review of the entire Veterans Health Administration program. His report described the VA as a "corrosive culture" in need of complete overhaul. One senator, Tom Coburn from Oklahoma, who had been a practicing physician and who had unappealing memories of working at VA facilities during his own medical education and training, had already launched an extensive investigation before the first reports of wait lists at the Phoenix VA. He found that the VA was riddled with incompetence and corruption.

Could it possibly have been that sanctioned delays of appointments were the only consequences of such a fundamental crisis in one of our nation's largest and most desperately needed federal programs?

Between 2003 and 2011, I was asked to lead a surgical program at one of the country's "best" VA facilities, the San Francisco VA Medical Center, as part of a joint appointment to the faculty of one of the country's top-ranked medical schools. By 2011 I had become a respected academician in the fields of molecular cardiac research and in the development of advanced systems for the treatment of lung cancer. I ran a research program funded by the National Institutes of Health. At the University of California, San Francisco, where I had my joint appointment, I had one of the lowest mortality rates of all the surgeons in my division, even though my practice focused primarily on very difficult cases that inevitably involved a higher risk of death and other complications. If, as was commonly believed at the VA, veterans represented a subpopulation of Americans with especially challenging healthcare needs, I seemed to be the perfect man for the job. But by 2011, I had learned that my disruptive demands for excellence were not going to be tolerated by VA administrators.

The most distressing aspect of the VA scandal of 2014 was the manner in which it was allowed to remain focused specifically on the delays of appointments. Once the American people, the media, and Congress began to penetrate the VA fog, they quickly demonstrated their deep concern for their country's veterans and asserted their right to know the truth—and their refusal to tolerate substandard care or abuse. Congress, anxious to appear decisive and effective, passed $16 billion legislation that promised little more than to speed up clinic visits, to allow the VA to hire more staff, and to sanction additional visits to non-VA practitioners. Remarkably, and despite the furor and the anger instigated by the wait list scandal, the country has now learned that the VA bungled implementation of the Veterans Choice program intended to fix just the waiting list problem. Nearly two years later, many veterans were waiting *longer* to be seen than they had before. And the VA budget has grown.

But what if waiting times at the VA were still just the tip of an ugly, disturbing iceberg of poor care, neglect, and abuse? As shocking as many of the 2014 revelations may have been, they pale in comparison to the true, appalling depth of abuse to which our veterans are routinely subjected at the VA. Just about any thoughtful medical academician who has worked at the VA could tell you that the VA wait list scandal of 2014 was nothing more than a reflection of the way everything is managed in that monolithic federal institution. And when an entire, badly broken healthcare system boils down to the generation and worship of a few dramatically misleading statistics, the disheartening result is not only a danger zone for our unsung heroes, but the violation of one of our nation's most important promises to a deserving, underserved population.

Recent revelations of continued failures in an expensive stopgap approach are bad enough. But it is time for American doctors and other healthcare professionals—people who have been aware of what the VA really represents and how our veterans are truly being treated— to force Americans to open their eyes to a much more fundamental failure of their government. A failure both to fulfill a promise and to remain accountable to the men and women who have already sacrificed so much for their country.

There is a great resistance in medicine to airing our own dirty laundry; the VA is a deep-set fixture in American medicine that very few care to rock. I actually began to collect my own notes of VA abuses after leaving my part-time involvement as the leader of a surgical subspecialty program at the San Francisco VA in 2011. Although I had begun to organize these notes even before the 2014 wait list scandal erupted, I was subsequently convinced to complete a memoir of my time at the VA. The following pages are the result of an effort to make sense of those notes and to put them into a larger perspective, a perspective that reflects back on the countless stories that have too quietly been told since the 2014 wait list scandal broke. I have interspersed among my own stories quotes from strikingly similar reports of VA abuses and failures from around the country, many of which were culled from Senator Coburn's scathing (yet largely neglected) report. It is my hope that this new, more comprehensive perspective will help shine a spotlight on unacceptable governmental abuse and ignite demands for truly meaningful change.

This book is based entirely on my experiences working within the Veterans Health Administration. That experience spanned twenty years and involved three separate facilities, each considered among the best hospitals in the VA system. All the events described in the book were real, but to protect the privacy of individual veterans and their families, the identities of all the patients have been disguised. The focus of this book is on the institution and not on the performance of any individual practitioners. The identities of all of the VA physicians have therefore also been disguised. I have identified Drs. Mark Ratcliffe, Brian Cason, and Diana Nicoll only in relation to their interactions with my own practice of thoracic surgery at the VA.

CHAPTER ONE

Edward Perry

The San Francisco VA Hospital's sprawling campus occupies a high hilltop rising above the western part of the city, some of the most expensive real estate in the United States. One side overlooks neat rows of homes in the city's Outer Richmond District; the other overlooks the bay and the stunning multicolored cliffs of the Marin Headlands.

A spectacular location. But if you don't have a car—and veterans in California often don't—it can be hard to reach. Vietnam vet Edward Perry was one of the carless. To travel from his home in northern California to the San Francisco VA, where I worked part of my time as a cardiothoracic surgeon, he had to take a series of uncomfortable VA shuttles. The trip began before dawn.

At least there were shuttles. If he'd taken public transportation, the trip would have lasted another hour or more each way. But VA transportation, even with help provided by Disabled American Veterans volunteers, could not afford to run direct shuttles from all over the region, or more than one shuttle connection each day; so the minibuses and vans from any distance out of town had to leave early if they were going to reach San Francisco by the start of clinics at about eight-thirty a.m.

I first met Edward Perry in early 2008 in my thoracic surgery clinic at the San Francisco VA. He was sixty-two, tall, lanky, leathery, craggy. Like so many vets we treated at VA hospitals, he was poorly dressed and rundown after a hard life of heavy drinking, heavy smoking, and physically demanding, poor-paying jobs.

"Hello, Mr. Perry. My name is Michael Mann." I always introduced myself at the beginning of an initial patient visit. It might have been the only way my patients could know they were actually being seen by their attending doctor, and not just by one of the VA's many residents and nurses. "I am one of the chest surgeons here at the San Francisco VA. I'm familiar with your case, and I've been studying your most recent scans."

Even before I stepped into the exam room, I already knew a good deal about Mr. Perry and the tortuous route that had led him to my clinic. A few moments earlier, my medical student, Rachel, had interviewed him. Rachel was a diligent, young apprentice from the highly regarded medical school at the University of California, San Francisco (UCSF), where I had my primary appointment. Before the interview, she had dutifully pored through Mr. Perry's medical record stored on the VA's electronic patient database, known as VistA. She had then briefed me in the clinic hallway outside the small room where Mr. Perry waited, while I took in his daunting radiographic studies on the hallway computer. Edward Perry had lung cancer.

As a thoracic surgeon, it was my job to operate on a variety of problems that crop up inside people's chests. Aside from a serious injury to the heart or the rupture of a massive blood vessel, lung cancer is the deadliest medical condition we face. An incredibly efficient killer, it now takes more lives worldwide than any other cancer, and in the United States it kills more people than the next four types of cancer *combined*. Just about the only way to survive beyond a few years after diagnosis is to cut it out before it has spread.

But only about a third of all lung cancers are picked up early enough to be operable, largely because most early stage lung cancers produce no symptoms. The other two-thirds of lung cancers have already spread to other parts of the body, or "metastasized," by the time they are diagnosed. For all of those patients, surgery is off the table. And even for the "lucky" ones with lung cancer who are eligible for surgery, the chances of survival are often no greater than 50 percent. In other words, you have to be very lucky.

In fact, the best way to survive lung cancer is to belong to an effective healthcare system that obtains CT scans of people's chests for a variety of reasons. In that way, doctors may find "early stage" lung cancers while they are looking for other things. But that healthcare system also has to be ready to jump on a finding of lung cancer and relentlessly prepare the patient for surgery while the time bomb of metastasis ticks. That means delivering the patient to a surgeon and performing an array of other tests that assess the extent of the cancer's spread, and whether the patient is in good enough shape to withstand a big, painful operation.

Mr. Perry's case was unusual, my medical student had explained. His relatively early cancer was discovered because it was actually making him cough. Unfortunately, the tough, stoic Perry was used to putting up with a lot more hardship than an annoying cough. The patient had ignored the symptom for some time. But, fortunately, he had a family, in particular a daughter, who noticed that his cough was different from the chronic hack that was a lingering reminder of the smoking her father had given up years before. Mr. Perry's daughter, Abby, cared a lot about her father and insisted on taking him to a local VA outpost, where a chest X-ray sent the family into a tailspin.

"I really appreciate your taking time to see me, doc," Mr. Perry said as I shook his hand. His positive sentiment was common among veterans in our clinics, even after their all-too-common long waits for treatment—waits that paradoxically made the doctors' time seem even more precious to the vets. Patients over at the university hospital often complained about "unreasonably" long waits that vets saw as normal and customary.

"It's been a long time getting here to see you," he continued, "a long time since this thing showed up. I know all those other doctors have been trying to help, but they seemed like they were mostly spinning their wheels. But you're gonna save me now. Right, doc?"

"In my line of work," I responded, knowing it was critical always to be honest with every patient, but also to inspire and nourish hope, "I can't make any promises, but we're going to do everything we can to get you past this tumor alive."

"I hope so, doc. That's what I've been waiting to hear."

We sat down in the chairs of my small, mostly bare exam room. An old, somewhat decrepit exam table stood against one wall, and an equally outdated metal desk was along the other. On the desk was a computer monitor and keyboard. Rachel stood quietly in a corner.

"My whole life," he continued, "I'da probably told you it didn't much matter whether my time was up or not. I lived my life like everybody else and didn't think life owed me anything. But now it's different, doc. That doctor who told me about this tumor on my X-ray told me that if a hundred people on the street came down with a lung cancer, only fifteen of them would be alive five years later. Shit, doc, I don't know nothing about math, but those numbers sound lousy. Five years is just not enough time for me. Not anymore."

"I understand completely, Mr. Perry," I said, hoping to gently steer the conversation toward the information I needed to know. "Your doctor was right. Lung cancers can be very tough." Training as a surgeon requires many skills that do not involve manipulation of scalpels and other instruments. Every physician must learn how to listen to patients, and to extract knowledge about their medical conditions that they may not even realize they have, information that could make an enormous difference in their treatment. But busy physicians and surgeons have limited time to spend with each patient, and so young doctors must learn how to guide their patients' narratives and make the transmission of information more efficient. I had hoped to direct Mr. Perry toward what I thought I wanted to learn from him. But as his story continued, something told me to listen to what *he* needed to say.

"I been hustled around these past six or seven months," Mr. Perry continued, undeterred by my attempts at redirection, "but if you're the man who's gonna cut me open and save my life, you gotta know why I can't just lay down and die. I lost my wife, Josephine, to breast cancer eight years ago. They told her she was stage four and put her through the chemo, and it didn't do much good. She was a wonderful woman, my Josie. I met her in high school, and she waited for me while they was fucking with my mind in Vietnam, and she stood by me all those hard years. I didn't deserve Josephine, that's for sure, and so I wasn't that surprised when she got taken away from me too soon.

"But now I've got Abigail, and everything is different. Abby was our only child, and what with her mom being so busy holding things together and then getting sick, and with me being so caught up in my own struggling to make it, we didn't give her the attention she needed, and she fell into a bad crowd. I always knew she wasn't like those other kids—real rough, no sense of right and wrong. But she got caught up with them, and we couldn't pull her out."

Mr. Perry paused. He wasn't short of breath, as are many pulmonary patients by the time they've gotten halfway through their stories, so much as short of energy. And probably short of hope.

"There was this one jerk," Mr. Perry said a moment later, staring at the floor in front of him, "who sorta took over Abby's life. Treated her like shit. But she thought he was gonna protect her. By the time she was twenty-two, she'd given him two little kids, Shaun and Kaitlin. Sorry, I got no pictures with me, but they're just the cutest couple of troublemakers you ever saw. Thank God, one day when he was drunk or high and about to get arrested, she realized she was worth something, too; and she grabbed the kids and made for the door and never looked back. Kaitlin was still in diapers. That was when I saw Abby had the fire I used to see in Josie's eyes. That's when I knew I was getting a second chance to deserve having those beautiful ladies in my life.

"Listen, doc." Mr. Perry's depression had given way to a sudden anxiousness. "Abby's got a good, steady job at the hairdresser's, and she's taking classes at night. She can't do all that and manage the kids by herself with the little she makes. In fact, I gotta sneak around and take the damn shuttles without her knowing 'cause I don't want her taking off from work just to bring me to these appointments. She's already taken too much time off to help me. She's gonna lose her job, and we'll be back to square one.

"I've got to be there now for the kids, doc. I gotta be their grandpa while Abby gets her life on track. Two or three or even five years is just not enough to make sure the kids have a home to go to and don't get into trouble like their mom. That wasn't her fault, it was mine; and now it's my chance to make it up to her. I don't want Abby feeling like she needs to find somebody else like that asshole who's gonna beat her up and mess up the kids. Abby needs her dad now, and I can't let her down.

"Doc, you can't let us down, either."

Even though I was riveted by Mr. Perry's story, I knew I had to get through my tutorial responsibilities, as well. I glanced furtively at Rachel, just long enough to catch the tears beginning to well in her eyes. This young doctor-in-training had learned a little about the patient's family during her routine interview. And in the hallway she had commented that it was strangely sad that Mr. Perry had come to see us all alone. Though she hadn't yet had much experience on the VA wards or clinics, she had observed painful discussions of life-threatening illnesses at the university, where families were almost always present to soften the blow. The young woman was perceptive enough to sense that Edward Perry was tremendously scared. And she had learned from him about how dearly he held his daughter and grandchildren in his heart. She seemed sad and a little angry that he did not now have a hand to squeeze as he faced a monumentally frightening choice. But she probably knew that for many of America's veterans, life had proved to be anything but easy after they returned from war, and that the legacy of those struggles often fell on their children. Both she and I sensed that if Edward Perry's daughter possibly could, she would have been there with him.

And that realization probably made Rachel even sadder and angrier.

After a brief but uncomfortable silence, I once again reassured my patient that if anything could be done to cure his cancer, he was in the right place and we were the right people to try. I had no reason to doubt that his mind had been "fucked" in Vietnam, or that his lifelong struggle to make it was at least in part a consequence of his military service. If those two things were true, his country may have owed him far more than he had received. It was my job to give him at least a partial payback.

I also wanted to make sure he understood the basics about lung cancer. He had undoubtedly heard most of it before, but he had to make an ominous decision. For that reason, I preferred not to take the chance that he faced that decision armed with less than the entire truth about his situation. Seven months earlier, a chest X-ray had suggested a "fullness" in the central part of his right lung. Based on Mr. Perry's age and significant history of tobacco use, the VA clinic doctor was immediately worried about lung cancer. A CT scan supported his suspicion.

At that point, there was good news and bad news. The good news: if the mass was a lung cancer, the scan also suggested that it had not yet spread. The bad news: this tumor, at 3.5 centimeters, was a bit large and located in a bad spot—at the root of the lung where major vessels and airways supplied all the blood and air to the rest of the lung. Removal of a tumor in that location often required removal of the entire lung, in an operation called a "pneumonectomy." Since people have two lungs, most patients survive a pneumonectomy; but the operation puts a significant strain on the heart and the remaining single lung. All the patient's blood must now pick up oxygen on that one side. Patients are more likely to die after a pneumonectomy than after the simpler and more common "lobectomy," where only one section of a lung is removed. The risks were especially high, as in Mr. Perry's case, when the cancer is in the right lung, the larger of the two; its removal leaves only the smaller, left lung behind.

Realizing he was in over his head, Mr. Perry's local clinic doctor quickly referred him to the regional center for lung cancer at the San Francisco VA. But the referral to the San Francisco Pulmonology Clinic had apparently gotten "lost." This was an unfortunate, but not uncommon, event. The cause could have been as simple as the referral being posted late on a Friday, with the Monday morning crew assuming that it had already been processed before the weekend. Less work for them. Regardless of the exact cause of the delay, and despite a recent VA dictum that all lung cancers be brought to the operating room within forty-two days of an initial abnormal X-ray, it was more than a month before the sheer persistence of Mr. Perry's daughter on endless telephone holds resulted in his finally being seen by my colleagues in internal pulmonary medicine at the San Francisco VA.

The doctors who saw Mr. Perry in pulmonology clinic knew exactly what to do. And realizing that they were both perilously close to the forty-two-day VA yardstick and losing precious time if Mr. Perry was to have a shot at survival, they tried hard to accelerate the remainder of his workup. He would need a bronchoscopy to confirm the diagnosis, a PET scan to look further for any spread of the disease, and a discussion of his case at the hospital's tumor board. The board would determine whether to send him straight to surgery or to send him first to a course of chemotherapy, with or without radiation treatments. The chemotherapy might reduce his chance of recurrence after the tumor was removed, and its combination with radiation might shrink the tumor enough to diminish the need for a pneumonectomy and allow the safer option of lobectomy.

Mr. Perry, however, was a patient at the VA, and that meant the process almost never moved smoothly or efficiently. Scheduling desks sometimes didn't seem to understand, or to care about, the significance of a doctor's request. Medical residents, with their incessantly rotating schedules, would most likely be the doctors who carried out plans and interpreted tests; they often did not realize the priorities that had gone into a patient's original diagnostic and therapeutic plan. Whatever the reason, it was two months before the relatively simple tests, obtainable within a week at UCSF, had been performed and the tumor board had referred Mr. Perry for preoperative chemotherapy and radiation.

At that point, Edward Perry's future took another dive. Once a patient is in the VA system, it is a painful, uphill struggle to persuade the institution to sanction care outside its four walls. Mr. Perry, however, lived too far from the San Francisco VA to make outpatient chemotherapy in San Francisco a reasonable option, and the San Francisco VA did not even have the technological capability to provide radiation treatment (for that, local vets were normally sent to UCSF). Although the tumor board had made a wise decision to recommend that local, private doctors near Mr. Perry's home provide this potentially lifesaving, preoperative treatment, which the VA would pay for, it was another month before the bureaucratic processing resulted in a single infusion of medication or a single beam of therapeutic radiation to Mr. Perry's chest. Another month of unchecked tumor growth. And another month for it to spread to a part of Mr. Perry's body where not even the most gifted surgical hands could remove it.

Six weeks of chemo-radiation were followed by another four weeks of waiting for a follow-up PET scan. These last four weeks were significant because there is a six-week window after completing radiation to safely perform surgery before radiation-induced scarring makes the surgery far more dangerous. Altogether, almost seven months had passed since Edward Perry's lung cancer had been seen on a routine chest X-ray. Luckily for the San Francisco VA, the "forty-two-day rule" went out the window as soon as his doctors had introduced the preoperative chemotherapy and radiation. In gathering performance statistics, the VA had determined that the "forty-two-day rule" would not apply when other courses of therapy were inserted between discovery of a lung tumor and its surgical removal. In this case, the chemo-radiation had been the right choice for this patient. But did it all need to take seven months?

This story was not what Mr. Perry needed to hear from me. He knew all that; he had lived through the nightmare of delays. What he needed to hear now was that his follow-up PET scan still did not show evidence of metastasis. That was good. In fact, it meant that his cancer was still potentially "operable." But whether the tumor had grown substantially before he received the chemo-radiation (and so was reduced back to close to its original size), or whether the therapy had just not been very effective, the tumor was not any smaller than it had been on the first CT scan, and so pneumonectomy was still the likely surgical choice.

And with that there were still unknowns: though his relatively large "early stage" lung cancer might still be curable with an operation, his chances of cure would go down from about 60 percent to about 45 percent if lymph nodes just outside the lung proved to be involved when they were examined after surgery under the pathologist's microscope. Perhaps more importantly, his complicated past medical history would make an operation more dangerous. Because he had a history of mild heart disease, a pneumonectomy might overstrain his already partially weakened heart. And because of a history of hepatitis and heavy drinking in the past, the patient had evidence of early cirrhosis in his liver. Depending on the severity of that disease, there could be an increased risk of bleeding and other complications.

I presented these possibilities for about five minutes with very little interruption from the older veteran. He hung on every word, knowing that this was where the months of painful therapies and painful delays had been heading. At the end of my presentation, I tried to sum things up so that he might have a fair chance to choose the hand he truly wanted to play.

"So, Mr. Perry, your other medical problems make any surgery riskier for you. There's an increased risk that there might be a lot of bleeding; there's an increased risk that you might have a big heart attack; there's even an increased risk that your left lung might fail or that you might get a serious infection after surgery. Any of those complications could take your life. Of course there are also always risks that we could injure something during the operation, and when we're operating in the chest, any injury could be life-threatening, as well. So if we decide to go after this cancer— and only you can make that decision—we've all got to have our eyes wide open. There's a chance you might not make it through. Now, based on your situation and our experience here, I'd say you're more likely than not to survive it. But then, with your stage of disease, there's also at least a 40 percent chance that the tumor's already spread and that it's already too late to cure you with this operation."

I could tell from his eyes that the veteran was paying extremely close attention to these words. He obviously understood what I was telling him.

"But without an operation, Mr. Perry, it's likely that this cancer will take your life. You might have a 20 percent chance of five-year survival with additional chemotherapy and radiation. Otherwise, it might take a year or two, or maybe three; it's unlikely to take more than that."

Those were the facts. I purposefully didn't muddy the situation with too many statistics. Complicated statistics hid the simple truth. There was a long pause before Edward Perry answered; I could feel the weight of his uncomfortable silence.

"Well, doc," he spoke at last, gazing again at the cracks in the exam room linoleum, "I know how busy you are, and I really appreciate your taking time to explain things to me. And I really appreciate your taking care of me, doc. I know you've got a lot of sick people to take care of, some of them sicker than me. Truth is, I don't really feel sick, at least I didn't before the damn chemotherapy. I hear you about the risks and all, but my daughter really needs my help, and her two little babies really need me, too. I've been feeling this thing inside me, doc, and it's not feeling good. Sure, I'm not sick, but there's something not right inside me, and it's getting worse.

"One or two years?" Edward Perry said, honing in on a stark conclusion. "Twenty percent? That's not enough. Mighta been before, but not now. You gotta help me lick this thing. I been in tight spots, and I never got out by worrying about the risks."

"I understand how you feel, Mr. Perry." For better or worse, I had built a practice, both at UCSF and at the San Francisco VA, that largely involved the types of cases that other surgeons, and other VA hospitals, avoided for fear of complications or bad outcomes. For those other doctors and institutions, nothing seemed like a better strategy for building a strong track record than avoiding situations where there was an inherent risk of disaster. And yet each of these tough cases was a human being with hopes, aspirations, and fears just like the rest of us. And with the same right to fight as the rest of us, and to have a clear picture of the odds and the nature of the looming battle.

"If you're willing to accept all the risks, you've come to a place where we take patients with these types of risks to the operating room all the time. We know how to do these operations. So now that we've decided to go ahead, all this talk of risks is behind us. Our whole team will be focused on one thing and one thing only: getting rid of your cancer and leaving the rest of you intact. We'll do everything possible to prevent complications, but we won't be obsessively worrying about them, and I don't want you to, either.

"I promise we'll take very good care of you. Unfortunately, I can also promise that there'll be pain. I'd be lying if I told you anything different. But it'll be our job to keep you as comfortable as possible after surgery so you can get up and get around as soon as possible. From now on, Mr. Perry, we're your team, and as far as I'm concerned, we've got just one goal: making sure you die of something besides lung cancer."

Nothing is more insidious than fear, either on the part of a surgeon or on the part of a patient. Like a cancer, it eats away at a person's psyche, undermining confidence and eroding the spirit and determination that keeps so many sick people alive until their bodies can recover. Once I've discussed risks and a patient has made a truly informed decision, I try to lessen fears and doubt in a patient and replace them with hope. Sometimes hope is the most important therapeutic element my operations bring to otherwise desperate and despairing patients.

Edward Perry's case was complicated both by a medical history filled with conditions that increased his risk of operative and postoperative complications and by the unnecessary delays that resulted from poorly organized and executed VA care. Not one incompetent doctor or nurse was to blame, but rather a system that was simply not driven by the expectation of excellence—or by accountability to it.

Instead of the normal two months of intensive preoperative therapy he would have received at most other hospitals, Mr. Perry came to my thoracic surgery clinic closer to seven months after his tumor was discovered. Despite the treatments, his tumor had continued to grow. And because of the sadly typical but unnecessary VA delays, his initially reasonable preoperative therapy had likely made it even more difficult for his body to survive an attempt at a surgical cure.

In the end, however, Edward Perry did not die from surgical complications. He never received an operation. Several days after our initial clinic visit, as I was rushing to place his case on my tight surgical schedule, I was informed by one of my administrative supervisors at the San Francisco VA that a right pneumonectomy was too high a risk in a patient who had undergone chemotherapy and who had Mr. Perry's combination of other serious medical problems. The VA, and our hospital in particular, had to limit the number of surgical deaths recorded in its annual statistics. Although Mr. Perry certainly would have been taken to the operating room and given a shot at survival at UCSF, and although his surgery had been recommended both by the San Francisco VA Tumor Board and by the hospital's Multi-Disciplinary Chest Conference, the administrator insisted on additional tests to document the patient's potential risks of cardiac and liver complications. Risks that we had no way of mitigating, risks that the patient had already recognized to be great when he provided a truly informed consent. During the further delays Mr. Perry encountered in scheduling these superfluous tests and evaluations, he contracted pneumonia as a result of the tumor that blocked his right lung. He had already been living on borrowed time, and the seriousness of his infection grew rapidly. He was admitted to the intensive care unit of a hospital near his home. He died there a few days later.

Edward Perry's death did not contribute negatively to VA postoperative mortality statistics. And his grandchildren are growing up without him.

* * *

Edward Perry was one of many vets who were not given a chance to receive high-risk but potentially lifesaving surgery at the San Francisco VA and at VA hospitals nationwide.

In fact, the San Francisco VA has been recognized as one of the best medical centers in the entire VA system. And by 2008, our hospital staff had grown accustomed to receiving blanket emails from our administration highlighting data that portrayed the Veterans Health Administration as the "best healthcare system in America," statistics that proved that the VA had superior "quality of care" and "patient satisfaction." Why then did Edward Perry fail to receive this superior quality of care? Why did we not save his life?

And why do so many other vets who trust the VA fail to receive the quality of care our nation has promised?

Over time, I realized that beyond this paradox was a more insidious connection between these very claims of superlative VA care and the deaths of patients like Edward Perry. Perry did not die from the high risk of his case. He was killed by an increasingly effective, systematic VA approach that limits the negative impact of high-risk cases on VA statistics, and therefore on the careers of VA administrators.

It was about the numbers. Limiting the number of deaths following surgery raised the rating of a VA hospital, and in so doing enhanced bureaucrats' careers (and annual bonuses). Without the need for any orchestrated conspiracy, decisions for or against surgery in particular cases were too often based not on the rights and wellbeing of the patients, but on the likelihood that surgical outcomes—outcomes that had at one time rescued the VA from harsh congressional scrutiny—would remain blemish-free. There was no need for conspiracy. It was simply the VA way.

Throughout the VA system in recent years, deaths following surgeries have been drastically, almost miraculously, reduced, just in response to heightened scrutiny. Why? Had surgeons' skills and the intricate coordination of complex care suddenly, spontaneously, and drastically improved? Or had people at the VA simply done what decades of box checking and obfuscation had taught them to do—game the system and make sure things looked the way people wanted?

Years after Edward Perry died, the nation was shocked to learn that dozens of VA hospitals had falsified waiting lists to overcome what had begun as an unreasonable bureaucratic demand to schedule every patient within two weeks. Yet no one has ever suggested an organized conspiracy. It wasn't necessary. Large numbers of VA administrators, doctors, and nurses had simply done things the VA way.

Mr. Perry lived and died the VA way. But what should have mattered more—bureaucrats' livelihoods or the lives of a veteran and his family?

Nearly 1,000 veterans' deaths have been linked to this kind of substandard care, with thousands of others impacted in similar ways at VA facilities around the country. Many cases involved patients suffering serious maladies, from hearing loss to mental illness to cancer.

–Coburn Report [2]

[As of June 2014], more than 20 veterans are dead or dying of cancer because they had to wait too long for diagnosis or treatment at just one VA facility in South Carolina. The deaths of three veterans at a VA facility in Georgia were caused by delays in care.

–Coburn Report [3]

Complaints of appointment cancellations, unanswered calls, and month-long waits make up a VA system that veterans describe as an "impenetrable and unresponsive bureaucracy." Many patients are lucky enough to turn to alternate health care coverage when the VA is unresponsive, but some veterans rely on the VA as their only option for medical care. Sadly, many veterans grudgingly accepted future

---

[2] In a 2014 oversight report, "Friendly Fire: Death, Delay & Dismay at the VA," then Senator Tom Coburn, MD (R-OK, 2005–2014) described numerous alarming facts that an investigation by his office had revealed about medical malpractice and neglect at the Veterans Health Administration. The report's findings are supported by more than a thousand factual references from VA facilities all over the country. This first excerpt is from page eight of the report.

[3] p. 8.

appointments because they felt they had no other choice.

—Coburn Report [4]

Claude V. D'Unger, a 68-year-old Army veteran from Texas, said he stopped seeking care through the VA after he was unable to timely schedule a CT scan of his lungs. "After calling for an appointment and being told that he would have to wait at least two months . . . he contacted a private doctor who performed the scan the next day." D'Unger also had problems getting in touch with people at VA clinics regarding his medical claims—someone rarely answered the phones when he called. "The claims side has a 1-800 number we refer to as dial-a-prayer," he said. "Nobody answers, nobody listens."

—Coburn Report [5]

---

[4] p. 13.

[5] p. 13.

CHAPTER TWO

Like Kissing My Sister

"Ι f I were in your shoes, I wouldn't be too excited about going out to the VA, either." The speaker was Dr. Nancy Ascher, one of the most accomplished women in American surgery and chair of one of the nation's most highly regarded departments of surgery, that of the University of California, San Francisco. She was referring, in the spring of 2003, to a plan for my initial appointment to her department's faculty, and also to the fact that she hoped I would agree to split my practice of cardiothoracic surgery between UCSF Medical Center and the nearby San Francisco VA Hospital.

Although the sentiment might have surprised many American laypeople and members of Congress who happened to have heard about the high quality of care achieved by the country's Veterans Health Administration, it would not have raised too many eyebrows among doctors trained in the United States, particularly not those involved in the pursuit of academic medicine. That's because nearly all of the physicians and surgeons who are trained in the United States spend at least part of their medical education or residencies at VA hospitals. They know firsthand what the place is like, and the types of career opportunities it does and does not provide.

Dr. Ascher's words, however, might have seemed to anyone like a curious way to convince me to agree to her plan, but that is exactly the type of person, and the type of leader, Nancy Ascher represented. Tough, bold, to the point. There was no bullshitting Nancy Ascher, and she would not waste time bullshitting you.

The point was simple: I was at the tail end of nine long years of surgical training—training that had started only after four years of college and another four of medical school. Tag on another five or so years of seeing the world and cutting my teeth as a director of biomedical research, and I was ready for my real career as a surgeon to finally begin. My scientific background was unusual for someone just coming out of residency, and therefore my prospects of successfully combining the practice of surgery with the conduct of molecular research were unusually high. That combination made me an attractive recruit to my own department at UCSF, where I had just been trained as a CT surgeon after completing my training as a general surgeon at Harvard's Brigham and Women's Hospital two years earlier.

I had wanted to be a heart surgeon for most of those seventeen years of higher education. During my training at UCSF, however, my admiration for the general thoracic surgeons, who operated on everything inside the chest *except* the heart, had drawn my interest to that sub-subspecialty, as well. Heart, or "cardiac," surgeons operate on, well, the heart, whereas most of general thoracic surgery involves the treatment of cancer. So these were two very different types of surgery, but, encompassed within the same body cavity, they had become connected at the administrative hip in American surgery, and every cardiothoracic surgeon trained in the United States has to pass a proficiency test in both. If my scientific background was unusual among newly trained CT surgeons, similarly unusual was my ongoing interest in actually practicing both.

Nancy realized that, after all those years of training and anticipation, I wasn't about to give up my chance to practice heart surgery on my own. But she also knew the lay of the land. Most Americans may view the practice of medicine and surgery as a highly refined, civilized, and compassionate component of our industrialized, market-driven society. Not necessarily so. In competitive urban areas like San Francisco, the practice of medicine and surgery is more aptly described as cutthroat than civilized. Scot Merrick, the chief of our Division of Adult Cardiothoracic Surgery and one of the last in my long line of mentors, gave me perhaps the most important lesson of my surgical training just as I was being sent out of the nest to wield a scalpel on my own. Scot was a tall man with an imposing presence, and his almost silent nature often suggested an air of quiet disdain; when he finally found a moment to say something, people listened.

"Remember," Scot told me one afternoon in the spring of 2003, "you will need the three A's if you're going to become a successful surgeon." The three A's, he went on to explain, were: availability, affability, and ability. Their levels of relative importance, he was quick to point out, were set firmly in that order. Most importantly, I would need to be *available*—not to patients, but to referring doctors, who were the gatekeepers and the source of all of a surgeon's practice and livelihood. Being available was a requisite to be sure, but it went nowhere if I couldn't then follow up my availability with an *affability* that would attract more of these internists' attention when they had additional patients to refer for surgery in the future. The *ability* to get their patients in and out of the operating room safely—and hopefully in better shape than when they entered—did make it onto the list of A's, but in Scot's estimation it was, unfortunately, a distant third to the other two.

Ironically, if I were to succeed as a heart surgeon at UCSF, I was going to need to take a slice out of a pie that was viewed much more as finite than expanding. And most of that pie belonged to Scot! Like other urban centers in the United States, the San Francisco Bay Area was blessed with numerous talented heart surgeons. But unlike many of those other highly desirable venues, where nearly all cardiac surgery was conducted at large academic centers, most of the heart surgeons in the Bay Area were "private slicks." And most of the heart patients were seen by private practice cardiologists, who had tight relationships with the private slicks. So the relatively anemic cardiology practice at UCSF could barely feed enough patients to Scot and the couple of other cardiac surgical mouths already at UCSF to keep them from hunger; the prospect of another mouth, no matter how exciting a "surgeon-scientist" it might belong to, was therefore a less-than-enticing prospect.

Still, Scot kept an eye on the big picture, and was a vocal proponent of my recruitment, recognizing the potential benefit of my appointment to our program beyond the implication of increased competition for himself. Joining Scot in support of my recruitment were the other leaders of our CT program: David Jablons, the chief of our division's Section of General Thoracic Surgery, and Mark Ratcliffe, chief of the Cardiothoracic Surgery Section and interim chief of the entire Surgical

Service at the UCSF-affiliated San Francisco VA. It was an unusual convergence of the stars; everyone wanted me on board. The problem was: Where would the extra heart surgery patients come from? It was not just a matter of my being bored—coming right out of training, I would need a rich experience of cases to build up my surgical skills and, more importantly, the surgical experience that would allow me to become a leader in my field.

But there was even more to the problem. While professors of history or English may be paid a salary directly from a university, the surgery faculty in medical schools almost always need to bring their own salaries to their departments through the collection of professional fees for their services. One of the reasons professors of surgery almost always earn significantly less than the private slicks, aside from allotment of a portion of their time to education and research, is that these professional fees go directly to their departments, where they are double or triple "taxed" by people like the medical school dean and the department chair. At the end of the day, surgeons are seen as cash cows, both for the academic medical center, which earns the highest margins on patients undergoing surgery, and for their medical schools and departments. Hiring a new guy with the explicit intention of spending half of his time away from the operating room (and away from revenue generation for the medical school and the hospital) is never a very popular proposal.

Like surgeons at HMOs, such as Kaiser Permanente, surgery professors are paid a salary by their departments. But the "allure" and "status" of the academic institution allows those salaries to be even less competitive than an HMO's. Still, that lower salary has to come from somewhere (it sure isn't coming from the medical school—money flows in the other direction). So for me, there would be both a shortage of experience building and a shortage of revenue generation at UCSF. Mark Ratcliffe, however, was eager to point out that over at the VA, he had a ready supply of both, just waiting for an up-and-coming young buck.

Mark was probably about the same age as Scot, but he looked at least ten years older. He was one of the few surgeons on the UCSF faculty who had agreed to be a full-time VA doctor, known as "eight-eighths" in VA parlance in reference to the full work week expected by the VA. For Mark, there was a very specific rationale: he viewed himself as a consummate surgeon-scientist. With a background in engineering, he had chosen to study the biophysics of the heart; he kept himself current and competitive by applying advanced computer modeling to the analysis of heart function and dysfunction.

Mark thought a lot about things—probably too much, which probably contributed to his premature aging. One of the things he loved to analyze was the predicament of a busy academic surgeon, trying desperately on the one hand to compete with private slicks to keep his medical center and department chair happy, while at the same time trying to compete with world-class scientists in the research arena who didn't need to trouble themselves with either private slicks or greedy deans.

Mark viewed the VA as the panacea for this predicament. The patients came in a steady supply, so there was no need to compete for them or even worry too much about how outcomes were perceived. A surgeon could forget about Scot's "three A's." It was a captive market that did not require any time or effort to cultivate. Unlike an HMO like Kaiser, though, the pace was slow and no one cared quite how many patients were gotten efficiently through the system. As long as it wasn't too few to justify a program's existence, a surgeon spending less time in the operating room made everyone at the VA happier. At the same time, the VA had claimed for itself a "research mission," and so part of a surgeon-scientist's VA time and salary could be openly apportioned to research. As financial pressures over the years made research funding from sources like the National Institutes of Health scarcer and harder to get than ever, and as competition and economics in the medical marketplace put more and more pressure on surgeons to be "productive" (i.e., generate revenue for the medical center), Mark became more and more convinced that the VA was a surgeon-scientist's utopia. He longed to prove this hypothesis, and he saw me as the perfect test case.

The final piece of my VA puzzle was that the San Francisco VA Hospital, viewed by many as one of the very best facilities in the national VA system, had been without a dedicated general thoracic surgeon to take care of lung cancer patients for at least two years. That was an obvious void for a system known to treat a population dominated by an elderly bunch of former and current smokers. The close affiliation of UCSF with their local VA made both Nancy Ascher and David Jablons somewhat responsible, together with Mark Ratcliffe, for filling this void. And so the scheme evolved: They all knew I was interested in maintaining an expertise in general thoracic surgery. I could, therefore, be parked part-time over at the VA and "put in charge" of general thoracic. Mark could throw a steady supply of cardiac surgery patients my way so that I could get my heart surgery career going without having to compete, at least not yet, with Scot or the others over at the university. My VA contract could have time built into it for setting up my laboratory and research program. And, last but certainly not least, the VA could pay a decent chunk of my salary, even as a part-time VA physician.

I should have been honored by the offer of leadership responsibility, coming straight out of residency. And yet, becoming the head of thoracic surgery at the VA felt a lot like kissing my sister.

I had had too much experience as a resident at VA hospitals (in Palo Alto, Boston, and most recently in San Francisco) to have illusions about the VA. VA hospitals were temples of mediocrity, where the practice of medicine was silently recognized to be somewhere below excellent. Most young doctors in the United States spend part of their residencies training at VA hospitals, and at the end of their residencies, most are thankful that they will never return. Nancy knew that, with ambitions to become a leader in my field, I would never agree to being full-time VA, but she and David were confident that my foothold in general thoracic at UCSF, together with an understanding that I would jettison the VA assignment at some time in the not-too-distant future, would be enough to seal the deal.

As usual, Nancy Ascher was right.

CHAPTER THREE

"Welcome Back"

I arrived at the San Francisco VA in the summer of 2003 with eyes wide open. After all, I already had more than ten years' exposure to the VA by the time my official tenure there as a staff member and program leader began. My earlier residency experiences at VA hospitals naturally reined in my enthusiasm for the renewed acquaintance. I had no delusions that I was joining a first-class medical establishment; if I had, Mark Ratcliffe, the man who had fought harder than anybody else to bring me there, made sure to dispel them soon after I arrived. One morning as we began to round on our mutual patients in the ICU, I wondered out loud why it always seemed harder at the VA to get additional cases scheduled in the OR, or to recruit dedicated thoracic anesthesiologists, or just simply to get things done.

"Michael," the prematurely silver-haired interim chief of surgery turned to me and said solemnly, "this is not the Cleveland Clinic."

Of course I knew he was right. I knew there would be mediocrity, resistance, and obstacles; yet I came on board confident that I would make a difference . . . if nothing else, then at least to the surgical disciplines for which I had been given specific responsibility. The shortcomings were all too familiar, but a handful of strengths in our program allowed me to be truly optimistic about what we might accomplish for the vets in San Francisco. I was determined to do everything in my power to drag cardiothoracic surgery and thoracic oncology up to or near the level of excellence in which I had been trained at UCSF.

Good luck to the VA if it tried to stand in my way.

Those intentions were quickly tested. One memorable event occurred during one of my first heart operations as an attending surgeon at the VA. It was a delicate and sophisticated procedure known as "off-pump" or "beating-heart" bypass. Traditionally, cardiac surgeons used an incredible invention of the 1950s and '60s known as a cardiopulmonary pump, or a "heart-lung machine," to allow the heart to be completely stopped during surgery. The patient's blood would be diverted away from the heart and lungs through a circuit of plastic tubing, replenished with oxygen, and then pumped back to the organs and tissues of the patient's body. As miraculous as this accomplishment was, doctors had known for many years that the circulation of blood through artificial tubing led to all sorts of hormonal and physiologic derangements in the patients after the operation was over. And so the concept of operating on the beating, pumping heart was revived from the pre-heart-lung machine era, and new, even more incredible technologies and techniques had been developed to make these "beating-heart" operations as safe and effective as the surgery that could be done "on pump."

If heart surgery sounds complex and somewhat mind boggling, it's because it is. In fact, a lot can go wrong during heart surgery. Years of training and repetition can prepare a CT resident for routine cases, but the mettle of any operating team is tested when things don't go according to plan.

I performed my first off-pump bypass as an attending at the San Francisco VA on a patient named Emerson Pitt, a navy veteran in his early sixties. At a critical moment during the procedure, and without taking my gaze off Mr. Pitt's beating heart, I extended my hand toward the scrub nurse and requested a two-millimeter coronary shunt. What I needed was a specially fabricated, tiny, silicon-tipped tube that I could insert into the two-millimeter diameter of the open coronary artery into which I was about to sew my bypass graft. The shunt would carry much-needed blood flow past the hole I had created in Mr. Pitt's coronary artery and on toward the heart muscle that was still pumping away and keeping him alive. Without the shunt, the heart muscle had even less blood flow than normal and was already beginning to struggle; it might not have lasted the ten minutes it would take me to sew in the graft.

"Shunt?" the nurse replied. "I don't have any shunts."

She was one of the regular nurses in the San Francisco VA cardiac OR, and so I had gotten to know her during the time I spent at the VA during my residency. She wasn't the type of scrub nurse who became part of the operation, the type of nurse I was used to working with over at UCSF. In general, UC nurses not only watched what was going on, they understood enough to anticipate what the surgeon would do next—and need next. I knew my VA scrub nurse that morning was not at that level of proficiency, but at least she had seemed fundamentally competent.

When something goes wrong during heart surgery, patients sometimes die. And sometimes, they die quickly. Solutions need to be fast and effective. I had just a few minutes that morning to come up with Plan B. Fortunately, I also had Marc Marcotte in the OR. Marc was a savvy, talented, and dedicated physician assistant. A rare VA gem—and smart. Smart enough to understand, without a drawn-out explanation, the plan I came up with to fashion a makeshift coronary shunt out of an ordinary intravenous catheter and some string.

Within a minute or so, he had the thing ready—and it worked. The rest of the operation proceeded smoothly, and Mr. Pitt not only tolerated the procedure well, but his heart thrived on the new blood supply brought by the bypasses. He recovered quickly from the operation and returned home five days later to his adoring family.

A handful of people like Marc Marcotte were some of the very elements that gave me hope about what we might be able to accomplish at the San Francisco VA. In fact, they were perhaps the most important reasons why I had agreed to launch my career there, at least in part. With Marc's help, a lot of effort, and a little luck, I believed we could be successful in raising the level of care for cardiothoracic patients at least a little higher than the typical VA standard.

On the other hand, a typically competent scrub nurse at UCSF would have alerted me to the absence of even a tiny but potentially crucial piece of surgical equipment prior to starting a case. But the blame for this particular failure certainly did not rest entirely with the VA scrub nurse that day; most of the failure, as usual, was with the VA. It turned out that the San Francisco VA had run out of coronary shunts a couple of weeks before during a similar "beating-heart" operation, and was not able to restock itself with the proficiency—or simple competence—expected of a modern American medical center.

∗ ∗ ∗

How had the VA developed into the type of organization that was so familiar to American doctors?

By the end of the twentieth century, the VA had become an entrenched part of American medicine. Though there were certainly variations in quality among VA facilities, there was also an unspoken attitude, comprised of impressions and expectations shared by VA doctors and other staff members, that was remarkably uniform across the system: fundamentally, the VA was a second-class institution that treated second-class patients. The attitude was unspoken, to be sure, but pervasive nevertheless. And it had developed in part out of the institution's haphazard evolution.

In fact, the history of the VA and its evolution into the largest, monolithic integrated healthcare system in the nation is almost as labyrinthine and confusing as many of the bureaucratic processes currently involved in its management. The Veterans Administration was officially created by Herbert Hoover in 1930, but the roots of the institution can be liberally traced back to 1636, just sixteen years after the Pilgrims landed at Plymouth Rock. Those early American settlers chose to provide pensions to colonists injured in battle with Native Americans. In 1776, the Continental Congress established a similar disability pension for the benefit of General Washington's injured soldiers. Pensions of one form or another then continued under the auspices of the federal government throughout the nation's history, but for many decades the actual care of disabled veterans remained the responsibility of states and local communities.

It was around the time of the War of 1812 that Congress decided both to build homes for former soldiers and sailors (although the first ones weren't built until decades later), and to provide pensions to veterans based on need, and not just strictly in compensation for combat-related disability. The focus remained on veterans who needed support, those who were down and out. When the Civil War brought the first real explosion in America's veteran population (from 80,000 to 1.9 *million*) Abraham Lincoln established a "National Asylum for Disabled Volunteer Soldiers." Its very name reflected an intention that it would provide a temporary helping hand to overcome transient adversity for those whose lives had been upended by war on an unprecedented scale. But by 1873, the names of the four existing facilities were changed from "Asylum" to "Home," and by 1884 eligibility was formally expanded to disability not only from war but also from age or disease. At that point, something more reminiscent of the modern Veterans Health Administration had emerged. "Homes" eventually evolved into hospitals, but a confusing system that patched together Pubic Health Service facilities, the Interior Department, and something called the Veterans Bureau persisted through a series of entanglements until Hoover brought all veterans services—medical, social, and financial—together under one administrative roof.

By the time a Department of Medicine and Surgery was finally established by the VA right after World War II, and its facilities were rapidly expanded to include 125 acute care hospitals, centuries of tradition, habit, and attitude had cemented people's impression of the VA as a safety net for the indigent victims of America's wars. This perspective and institutional attitude persisted and became indelible, and inevitably influenced the expectations of nearly everyone involved in its provision of care. Doctors from nearby medical schools were heavily recruited as part-time staff, enticed by the promise of vast numbers of patients who could service the needs of their students and trainees. VA care was a handout; it was not a noble obligation borne by the nation to an honored segment of society. To the contrary, the vets who availed themselves of the VA were perceived for the most part as unsuccessful members of society; whatever the VA could provide to them was better than nothing.

By 2003, when I joined the ranks of part-time VA physicians, the VA had been transformed once again, this time by Ronald Reagan and George H. W. Bush into a cabinet-level Department of Veterans Affairs. Its annual budget of more than $60 billion comprised one of the largest single-ticket items in the US federal budget. The San Francisco VA "Hospital," where I would spend at least thirty-five hours of my typically eighty-hour workweek, was actually an expansive complex perched atop a hill overlooking the Golden Gate Bridge to the north and the Pacific

Ocean to the west. The inpatient hospital and outpatient clinics comprised only a very small portion of the total real estate involved, which encompassed more than twenty buildings ranging from a plethora of administrative offices to animal research facilities. In addition to the many administrative offices, there were also a few specialized treatment centers (including a small psychiatric facility), and even a small long-term care unit akin to a nursing home. There was a large and varied staff, although only a minority seemed to be involved directly in the care of patients. The rest took care of paperwork, conducted basic science and clinical research, administered the research programs, and provided support to other facilities. The inpatient hospital was actually relatively small, with fewer than 150 acute care beds, modest for its role as a regional provider of complex, tertiary medicine.

I had encountered many VA shortcomings like the missing coronary shunt during my residencies at VA hospitals. I would encounter many others—and worse—over the ensuing years. Yet, the shunt incident in no way moved me to abandon my hopes for improving practices at the VA. In fact, it shone a light on one of my chief reasons for maintaining hope: the presence within the system of a few sharp, talented, resourceful, and conscientious people, people like Marc Marcotte. And people like Michael Baker, the OR nurse who had been assigned to organize our new effort at establishing a proficient general thoracic operating room. Michael was roughly six feet tall with somewhat of a barrel moustache, and he had a pleasantly optimistic way of approaching his work. He pointed out to me more than once that he had come from a humble background and that he had worked hard to make a better life for himself as a registered nurse. He was profoundly confident that his common sense and his dedication could overcome any deficits in his more formative education and training. And he was determined to do his best to help me create a world-class thoracic surgery program where there had been none.

"Have we gotten any of that new mediastinoscopy equipment?" I asked Michael one day during that early period of program building, referring to the replacement of a group of specialized general thoracic instruments. The ones I had come across in the San Francisco VA OR looked very little like the state-of-the-art equipment on which I had been trained over at UCSF. Instead, they looked more like World War II surplus, or pieces on loan from a Smithsonian exhibit on the history of surgery.

"You've got to be kidding, Dr. Mann," Nurse Baker responded with a smile. "I've been tracking down the vendors and order numbers, but our catalogues seem to be out of date. I've got a call in to the people over at UC to see what they have and where they got it."

That all seemed reasonable, but Michael went on, clearly hoping to temper expectations.

"But I wouldn't hold my breath for too long. Even if I figure out what we can get, there's a lot of red tape between us and those instruments, Dr. Mann. Remember, this is the VA."

∗ ∗ ∗

But the true patron saint of San Francisco VA cardiothoracic surgery was an indefatigable nurse by the name of Dallis Manwaring.

Dallis, who fulfilled the role of a nurse practitioner (although she did not technically have the full qualifications) and whose job it was to help organize and manage our VA's Cardiothoracic Surgery Service, had dedicated her life to serving the often otherwise underserved men and women who passed through the San Francisco VA. Nurse Manwaring had been at the VA for ages and knew all of its peculiar ins and outs. Most importantly, she knew exactly where things would get held up and screwed up, and she was therefore often the only one who could get things done. Marked by her insuppressible grin, and a slightly subdued effervescence, she was as dedicated to the wellbeing of every one of her patients as any health care professional I had ever met. And she was determined not to let the VA stand in her way.

Though too many on the hospital staff worked at the VA for no better reason than convenience and apathy, I did perceive, in general, a measure of compassion for the vets as individuals. As a collective group, however, the vets were often perceived as second class. But some, like Marc and Dallis, stayed on at the VA out of a deep commitment to and respect for the veterans. They adapted to the VA environment, and they developed ways to defeat the inertial and counterproductive aspects of the system.

There were a few other encouraging elements at the VA during those early years. One was certainly the significant number of world-class doctors from UCSF who rotated through. During a rapid expansion of the VA after World War II, a plan called for each hospital to collaborate with a nearby academic institution, if one was available. The medical schools provided faculty to help staff the VA (raising the average caliber of its doctors), and the VA provided additional patients who were often readily available to participate in clinical research projects and in the schools' education programs. The San Francisco VA, however, had developed especially close and substantial ties with UCSF. Every doctor at the San Francisco VA had to have an academic appointment at UCSF, even those who were full-time VA. Many great physicians and world experts spent time at this sister campus. One enticement the VA offered was facilities for the abundant, cutting-edge research led by UCSF faculty members, facilities that were always scarce at UC's confined, urban campus.

There were also ubiquitous reminders of an official VA policy that at least paid lip service to the concept of quality improvement. This policy generated an inviting atmosphere for open discussion that sometimes even produced positive results. One concrete example was the response of the Multi-Disciplinary Chest Conference (the so-called MDC) to my arrival as a dedicated general thoracic surgeon. Having been reared on the sophisticated Thoracic Tumor Board at UCSF, which was a regular meeting of true world experts who discussed challenging cases that came through the UCSF clinics, I was eager to help recreate some of the highly erudite, academic give-and-take that always seemed to benefit the diagnostic and therapeutic plans for our university patients. Before long, cases that had previously been rejected as hopeless at the San Francisco VA were being considered by the MDC for new, cutting-edge approaches. Tired, old preconceptions were being challenged by new clinical data. Although we could never claim the full breadth of specialists at this MDC that we enjoyed at the UCSF Thoracic Tumor Board—we had no pathologists, for example, and no specialists in radiation therapy—attendance and interest levels both rose considerably as the months and years rolled by.

And with it all, there was Mark Ratcliffe. Mark both managed the cardiac side of things and was a serious biomedical researcher, but more importantly, he had earned my loyalty and trust through his unbridled backing during my recruitment to the institution. Soon after my arrival, he followed through on his promise that my VA "tour of duty" would reflect a healthy mix of patient care and research. Although I was just off the blocks, as Mark would put it, as a fully fledged surgical attending, my research had brought me to a junior faculty appointment at Harvard even before my general surgery residency had been completed. Academic surgeons of the twentieth century had been known for their prowess as researchers of physiology, but by the turn of the millennium, understanding organs had given way in the medical scientific community to understanding molecular biology and genes. I was an unusual surgeon in that I was trained in and had led sophisticated molecular genetic research, research that had already made the challenging transition into the testing of new, molecular human clinical therapies.

In his unwavering support, Mark not only provided me with a generous amount of well-equipped research laboratory space on the VA campus, he also secured a seed grant of $75,000 from a research foundation affiliated with the San Francisco VA to help get my laboratory work back off the ground. He and I frequently spoke about our rescarch and about our patients, and he frequently discussed with me in confidence difficult aspects of his job, and even the colorful personalities he had to contend with both at the VA and over at UCSF. Most importantly, Mark was eager to become my mentor, and I felt lucky to have that level of support from the top of our VA surgical department.

I was not only the newest cardiac surgery attending at the hospital, but also the new guy in charge of general thoracic surgery. For the next eight years, I would call myself the "head" of general thoracic surgery at the San Francisco VA. Although I was clearly put in charge of non-cardiac thoracic surgery, and was given full responsibility for reviving and maintaining that neglected specialty at the institution, I was never given the authority nor the resources of a true "section chief." Instead, general thoracic surgery was lumped together with cardiac surgery as a "Cardiothoracic Section," of which Mark Ratcliffe remained in charge until the last few months of my tenure there.

But in 2003, I was finally on my way. I just didn't know where I was headed.

CHAPTER FOUR

"Remember, This Is the VA"

The VA wears you down.

When you walk into a VA hospital, you don't always see the kinds of patients you see at most private American hospitals. Many of the vets treated at VA hospitals are poor; some of them are not so well dressed, not so well put together. Many have lived difficult lives, and it shows in their bearing and in the way they walk. They are not used to expecting or demanding the best. They are grateful, most of the time, if they are handed second or maybe even third best. They are generally very grateful for whatever they get at the VA; they are particularly grateful to get it for free.

The attitude of the vets toward the institution and the attitude of the institution toward the vets are in sync. The collective, perhaps unconscious, attitude of the institution assumes that whatever it provides is basically good enough. Sometimes, individual providers do strive to reach a level of excellence that they are used to at other institutions, but they inevitably accept "reality" when other elements of the VA machinery make that truly excellent care more difficult, or sometimes "impossible," to achieve.

This unspoken attitude applies to nearly everyone in the institution—from the maintenance staff up through the doctors and administrators. It wasn't, for example, obvious to me and to other VA doctors that we shared such an attitude toward the vets, or that it influenced our expectations of what we needed to accomplish on their behalf. But we did share it. And that was precisely because the attitude was so effectively pervasive: these were the "vets."

In fact, when I looked back at my early years on staff at the VA, I realized that the place had me coming and going. When people first step into a position there, they are immediately drawn in to a prevailing attitude, an unspoken and yet absolutely unquestioned "truth" that engulfs their minds and becomes their adopted reality. I had no idea at the time that I, too, had been pulled in by an undertow of prejudice and was mired in a sea of assumptions that inevitably would impact my attitudes, perceptions, and even my professional decisions.

I didn't realize that until much later.

What was that unspoken "truth"? Simply put: the vets were second-class patients, representatives of our society's lower echelons, and often of the downtrodden or even the down-and-out. The direct corollary of that truth was that they were lucky to get whatever they could from the VA. And the direct and unfortunate corollary of that unspoken belief was that the mediocrity of the VA was therefore just fine for many of the staff who had come to work at the VA with the understanding that expectations of them would not be high. And if mediocrity was not "just fine" for those of us who did aspire to much higher standards in other parts of our professional lives, *VA mediocrity* was at least an acceptable (and unavoidable) compromise during our time within that particular institution.

If the vets were "second class" because of our perception of their general socioeconomic status, it was also an unquestioned "fact" throughout the institution that vets were "sicker" than patient populations at "normal" hospitals. Because of the stress of their hard lives and their frequent poverty, they had more complicated medical histories and more numerous and more advanced medical problems than the "average" American patient. Of course, their outcomes would therefore inevitably be worse than "normal" or "average" patients'. That attitude led directly to a greater acceptance of poor outcomes and a broad lowering of expectations, even among part-time VA physicians like myself who would consider such expectations unacceptable at our home institutions.

Our view that the veterans were a more challenging patient population could have engendered a determination to work even harder at the VA, to overcome the additional challenges that the veterans' socioeconomic conditions bestowed upon their medical care, and to live up to the national promise of the VA by bringing the vets' medical conditions more in line with the average American's. Unfortunately, no such determination materialized. Instead there was a simple acceptance of the "reality" that the vets were—and always would remain—a sicker bunch.

Another result of the impression that vets were generally less healthy than their peers was a bizarre, almost comic corollary conclusion: their survival in the face of all of these adversities led to the running half-joke that vets were "indestructible." Nearly all practitioners at the VA have joked, at one point or another, that "you can't kill a vet, they're tougher than nails." Of course, needing to struggle, as many of them do, against real disadvantages has helped many of them to develop a toughness and a determination to persevere. But this half-joke only promoted the unfair, deleterious, and prejudicial perception that the veterans of our armed forces were a distinct patient population and that it was acceptable to harbor a distinct set of expectations for their care.

Another unquestioned VA "reality" was that this was not a place where the best medical resources could be found. Mark Ratcliffe was right: this "was not the Cleveland Clinic." This particular attitude had become self-fulfilling. As the decades passed, and as the VA became established in people's minds as a second-rate institution that treated second-rate patients, it attracted, in general, a segment of the medical profession (at all levels, from orderly to chief of staff) who were driven by lesser motivations than the drive for professional excellence.

It was not that all VA employees were incompetent or lazy, or that there were no incredibly talented, hardworking individuals at the VA. Certainly there were. But every VA employee was affected by an *institutional* laziness, institutional assumptions about what could and could not get done. Even when VA initiatives and congressional appropriations led to updated equipment and facilities, these entrenched attitudes and assumptions remained. If acceptance of reduced pay and reduced professional self-esteem was associated with a career at the VA, there had to be some benefit in return. A quid pro quo. For many—not all, but many—it was the promise of a slow and comfortable pace of work, an environment where checking boxes would fully meet professional expectations and where demands for outstanding performances just did not exist.

For those few who remained committed to achieving the best possible care for their VA patients, the institutional laziness meant that *their* work would be even harder and more exhausting.

> Two out of three intensive care unit staffers at the Lexington, Kentucky VA conceded they 'would not feel safe being treated as a patient' at the facility, and 'high percentages of staffers in other departments gave the same response.'
>
> –Coburn Report [6]

Of course, at some level I was consciously aware, as were all my colleagues from UCSF, that the vets were not getting what we would be capable of delivering to them at the university. And I never fully abandoned my hopes and intentions to raise the bar for the care that would be provided to my patients at the VA. But the VA wears you down. It's the passive inertia, and it's the active resistance. My hopes and dreams gradually, imperceptibly faded in the face of obstacles, mediocrities, frustrations, and frictions that were a natural consequence of VA traditions and culture. At the VA, doing it well lost out to simply getting it done.

That is, when we could get it done. One incredible paradox of my time as a cardiothoracic surgeon at the San Francisco VA was the perpetually long list of patients waiting for heart surgery versus our struggle each week to fill our four skimpy cardiac surgery slots on the operating room schedule. Four heart surgeries per week, at what Mark Ratcliffe claimed was the best surgical VA hospital in the entire system. One case per day, four days per week—with one entire day off from operating just so that one of the three or four cardiothoracic surgeons could attend a half-day clinic. Busy cardiac surgery programs in private hospitals in the Bay Area might have gotten four cases done *per day*. But the few times

---

[6]   p. 10.

I suggested getting two cardiac cases done in a day at the San Francisco VA, and the fewer times still that I actually pushed hard to do it, I might as well have been suggesting to light a bonfire in a propane gas factory.

Our inefficient handling of cardiac surgical candidates was not entirely for lack of trying. Once every week, the VA cardiothoracic surgeons, the CT chief resident, and Dallis Manwaring, our nurse coordinator, all sat down around a long conference table in the surgical offices for the Cardiothoracic Service meeting. When I had been a trainee on the service, those weekly meetings had seemed primarily aimed at testing both the residents' familiarity with each of the patients and the residents' working knowledge of how each one needed to be treated. Shortly after my transition to the faculty, however, my perspective changed. The meeting now seemed to provide a much-needed opportunity for the attending cardiothoracic surgeons to review each of the many cases on our operative waiting list, and also the several patients who were inevitably vegetating on our postoperative wards. The conference was no longer an intensive educational exercise; it was an administrative tool intended to manage a service that often seemed on the brink of dysfunction.

A typical service meeting often began with a discussion of the complications and unanticipated turns that kept some of our post-op patients in the hospital longer than expected.

"Mr. Kominsky?" Mark Ratcliffe asked of his team one morning. "Why is he still here? I thought we were sending him to a SNF."

Prolonged hospital stays increased patients' risks of hospital-related complications, not the least of which were infections with super-resistant bacteria that are routinely found in acute care hospitals. But in addition to the theoretical advantages of discharging a patient as soon as possible, there was a clear administrative advantage to getting patients off of our service and into skilled nursing facilities (the acronym for which was pronounced "sniff"). VA cardiac surgery statistics were heavily influenced by the occurrence of death or serious complications within thirty days of an operation. If a patient made it past the critical thirty-day mark, but remained in the hospital, a death or complication before discharge still counted in the all-important thirty-day statistics. Once day thirty rolled around, it was imperative to get the patient out the door—even if there was a good chance of rapid readmission.

"He was teed up to leave," the resident began to explain, "but then his blood sugars shot through the roof. We consulted endocrine and even put him on an insulin drip [a constant infusion of insulin through an intravenous catheter], when finally we realized he was scarfing down the regular Jell-O, ice cream, and other deserts that were being delivered to his room on his *non-diabetic* food trays."

Mark just shook his head. This was far from the first time that any of us had wandered into a diabetic patient's room at the VA and found packets of regular sugar and other sugar-laden delicacies, despite the doctors' orders clearly stipulating a diabetic, sugar-free diet.

"Fortunately," the resident continued, "we picked up on the high blood sugars before he had a chance to go into ketoacidotic shock."

"Yeah," began Mark's only comment on the subject, "Mr. Kominsky was really fortunate."

After a few moments of uncomfortable head shaking, as the attendings avoided each others' gazes by looking down at the patient lists sitting on the long table in front of them, Mark piped up again.

"That reminds me," he continued, "did they ever find Mr. Jackson?"

Arnold Jackson was a veteran of Operation Desert Storm who suffered with a complex of symptoms that fell under a poorly characterized and even more poorly understood phenomenon known as "Gulf War Syndrome." Mr. Jackson was also an intermittent IV drug abuser, and his use and reuse of unsterile needles had led to an infection of his heart valves known as "endocarditis." His homelessness didn't make the many weeks and months of his required antibiotic treatment any easier, and he had therefore spent a lot of time at the San Francisco VA.

Finally, after having received an adequate, though frequently interrupted, course of intravenous antibiotics for his infection, he had been brought to the operating room for replacement of the damaged, leaky valve in his heart. Surgery had gone reasonably well, and in consultation with the Infectious Disease Service, it had been decided to continue two more weeks of postoperative intravenous antibiotics to minimize the risk of recurrent infection of the patient's new valve.

So Mr. Jackson was on an ordinary ward, recovering from a painful splitting of his breastbone, but he was otherwise in relatively decent shape. He had always been prone to transient periods of disorientation, but they were infrequent and of limited duration. Two days before this particular service meeting, however, when the cardiac surgery team descended to Mr. Jackson's floor on afternoon rounds, the patient was nowhere to be found.

To be sure, these were not locked wards, and patients had the right to refuse care at any time, and even to leave the hospital "AMA" (another acronym that meant "against medical advice"). But we at least wanted to know when a patient was considering such a move. We certainly needed a chance both to talk things over and to make sure an unsatisfied patient had all the facts and was as well prepared as possible for what might lie ahead, especially given the particulars of a likely complex medical problem. We certainly did not expect our patients simply to disappear.

To be sure, the VA nurses were not security guards, and they had numerous responsibilities that occupied their attention. A savvy, stealthy patient likely could not be stopped from sneaking off a ward unnoticed. But Mr. Jackson, particularly in his less lucid moments, could not be described as either particularly savvy or stealthy—loud and disruptive was more likely. And so it was not terribly unreasonable for us to expect a patient like Mr. Jackson to be stopped when wandering off during a fit of disorientation, at least for him not to make it very far in his hospital garb before some member of the staff came to his assistance.

There were several particularly problematic aspects of Mr. Jackson's disappearance. Of course, he wasn't getting his intravenous antibiotics. Even more concerning, he had an IV in his arm that was not only at risk for a new infection—now even more dangerous with a new, artificial heart valve in place—but the IV itself was a beautifully built-in portal for further intravenous drug abuse. The potential double whammy of a dirty syringe being plugged into the IV for that purpose was particularly disturbing. But being out and about around the VA campus (or worse yet on the city streets) with nothing more than his hospital clothes and no resources for self-care was just too dangerous a situation for us to accept for an early postoperative patient like Mr. Jackson. On a more fundamental level, we felt completely responsible for our patients' care and well-being until they were ready for discharge after major, life-altering, and life-threatening surgery. Losing them just did not seem consistent with that imperative. Nor did it seem like good medicine.

> The IG [Inspector General] found various flaws in several management practices at the Miami SARRTP [Substance Abuse Residential Rehabilitation Treatment Program] that enabled a patient's fatal overdose. The report noted insufficient patient monitoring and supervision, including defective surveillance cameras and lax contraband searches when patients returned from pass outings. The IG also discovered staff members were not always physically present at the SARRTP unit as required, and patients who leave the facility enjoy easy access to illicit substances due to the facility's location in a high-drug area.
>
> –Coburn Report [7]

Mr. Jackson was found about eighteen hours after we discovered his disappearance. It was unclear how long he had been gone before that. The VA police had begun to search our surrounding neighborhood. Unfortunately, this wasn't the first time that our neighbors had been alerted to a patient's disappearance and that their assistance in locating a missing patient had been enlisted. He was found on a street corner not far from the VA complex and brought back to his ward to complete his two weeks of postoperative antibiotics.

Mark was given this bit of good news about Mr. Jackson, and we then turned our attention to the surgical waiting list, and to a discussion of the sticky heart valves and clogged up coronary arteries that should have already been fixed in the operating room, but for one reason or other still remained mired on The List. The List was always dozens of patients long, and yet, week in and week out, it remained a challenge to fill up the four available OR slots with patients who were fully ready to go. Some patients needed additional tests that would take weeks to schedule, only to be cancelled with or without the patient ever having been informed. Some patients needed to wait to see specialists

<hr>

[7] p. 11.

for unrelated problems that might conceivably make their surgeries more dangerous. Other patients were just plain hard to reach, and when someone as perseverant as Dallis finally got them on a hallway phone in a vagrant hotel or at a homeless shelter, there would be some other obstacle preventing us from whisking them into the operating room, where they needed to be.

Dallis seemed able to juggle the entire List in her head, and she would update us regularly on every confusing wrinkle that kept almost everyone on The List from being ready for surgery. But despite Dallis's uncanny mastery of The List, the delays never ceased; some vets inevitably suffered as a result.

> Veterans "experienced excessive wait times" at the North Texas Veterans Health Care System. At least five patients referred for vascular access had to wait three months or more for a procedure, with one dialysis patient waiting for "more than 4 months for permanent vascular access." Ambulatory monitoring for a cardiac patient was delayed three months, while more than 200 others scheduled for ambulatory cardiac monitoring waited an average of 68 days. The clinicians "did not review referral requests, consultation reports were not linked to requests in the HER [Electronic Health Record] as required, and appointment dates requested by patients for vascular and cardiac procedures were incorrectly recorded by scheduling staff."
>
> –Coburn Report [8]

The career interests of the attending surgeons themselves would sometimes come into conflict with the patients' needs. The composition of our group of surgeons changed over the years, but on the surface, we

---

[8] p. 13.

all probably seemed fairly similar. Each of us had an Ivy League background of some sort, and each of us had chosen to go into "academic" medicine—to become teachers and/or researchers at an institution of medical education, rather than pursue more comfortable and lucrative careers in private practice where all one did was operate. Despite there being some component of altruism in that decision, there was also a demand on each of us to maintain academic "productivity." That demand could result in a significant degree of pressure for us to complete research programs and other projects outside of our already busy clinical schedules, especially since we all had to advance academically in the extremely competitive environment of a high-powered university where many professors did little more than conduct research.

And along with the acceptance of and expectations for poorer outcomes came an equally insidious perception of VA patients as an available "commodity" for the doctors' various professional needs. Residents could exploit a special training experience, and were able to "take more charge" and to make more "independent decisions." Faculty members used this same excuse to delegate more of their own responsibility (and sometimes their work) to their residents at the VA, allowing the professors sometimes to limit the same residents' exposure to their "more valuable" "private patients" at the university. For some doctors, VA patients remained a ready, captive source of increased "volume" for their own professional development. Some felt they could more easily recruit patients for research programs; some surgeons even felt they could more easily try out new or unfamiliar techniques. If a VA patient had to wait for the convenience of an attending physician's schedule, that was much easier to swallow than at our outside practices. Although people still tended to interact politely and often compassionately with each individual patient, the veterans as a group were commoditized; they were there for us as much as we were there for them. No one was going to steal them away, and they weren't going anywhere on their own.

Sure, strict rules protecting patients' rights were in place at the VA, just as they were at UCSF and any accredited hospital in America. But, unlike the "private" patients at UCSF, the vets were used to being scheduled for care without much of their own input. Their surgeon was chosen for them, either by the day they happened to be plugged into Cardiothoracic Surgery Clinic, or by the vagaries of the scheduling done at our weekly service meeting. More than once, a surgery scheduling decision for a particular patient was delayed because an attending really wanted to do the case a certain way, and was only available to do it on a certain day or a certain week. Sometimes that certain way seemed a little more complicated—and a little more dangerous—than absolutely necessary to the rest of us, but it was an unstated understanding that the surgeon involved really wanted more opportunities to enhance his or her career development.

At this particular meeting, one of the attendings indicated to Dallis that exactly such a scheduling change needed to be made.

"We've gone over this before," Dallis began after taking a deep sigh. In the end, Dallis actually took responsibility for everything that needed taking care of on the Cardiothoracic Surgery Service, and when she was pushed too far, she ceased to beat around the bush. "Mr. Heinrichs and his wife have already struggled to make arrangements to get his surgery done this Monday. They've got cousins coming in from Arkansas over the weekend to help manage their business. I must've spent thirty hours on the phone helping to arrange for medical leave from their jobs in Arkansas. This is not—"

"I know, Dallis," the attending surgeon interrupted, unmoved by Dallis's exposition. "You're a miracle worker. I know you can get all this rearranged for the seventeenth."

It took Dallis a few seconds to realize the implication of this new demand.

"That's two weeks away! Mr. Heinrichs has already been waiting for three months to get on the schedule. His wife called yesterday to let me know that his chest pain and his shortness of breath are getting worse!"

"Why has he been waiting for three months?" one of the others around the table chimed in, likely out of both curiosity and a desire to defuse some of the growing tension.

"He needed a new echocardiogram," Dallis began after yet another long sigh that intimated that she had probably provided this answer at least a half-dozen times before at similar meetings. Regardless, we had all heard similarly pathetic explanations for similarly unjustifiable delays of care at this institution many more times than any of us cared to remember.

"One of our echo techs has been on disability leave with carpal tunnel," Dallis continued, "so the echo lab has been down to one tech and it's been impossible to get anyone onto their schedule. Then we decided that Mr. Heinrichs also needed to be scoped by the GI service because there was some question as to whether he had ever had a GI bleed."

Some patients have a tendency to bleed internally. Those patients could have a nasty complication if they undergo heart surgery. A real history of internal bleeding, therefore, needed to be taken seriously and investigated thoroughly before any operation on the heart. But over the years, we seemed to become more and more averse to the impact of complications on our service's cardiac surgery statistics. And so it had been decreed that every patient with even a slight suggestion of ever having had a GI bleed of any magnitude needed to be examined by the gastrointestinal doctors just to make sure that their risk of a bleeding complication would be low. That meant colonoscopy (i.e., having a very long black tube with fiber optics pushed up through the patient's anus and run all the way through the large intestine).

"But you know the GI guys also complain about being constantly overbooked," Dallis went on, "and they also don't like to do these high-risk cases." As one can imagine, the experience of colonoscopy can strain a patient's heart—exactly what someone with a heart like Mr. Heinrichs's needed to avoid. "And so they refused to even schedule him for colonoscopy until we were certain he was a surgical candidate."

"And did he ever get scoped?"

"Of course he did." At that point, the exasperation seemed to be welling up in Dallis's throat. "But we couldn't even schedule the colonoscopy until the echo had gotten done!"

Dallis took a moment to regain her composure.

"So now it's been three months, and Mr. Heinrichs, with his tight coronaries, is kind of a walking time bomb."

"He's been fine for years." The last word on the subject often followed this definitive, often self-evident truth. "He can wait another week or so."

In 2011, Edward Laird, a 76-year-old Navy veteran, noticed two small blemishes on his nose. His doctor at the VA hospital in Phoenix ordered a biopsy, but as months passed, he was unable to get an appointment. After filing a formal complaint as his blemishes continued to grow, Laird saw a specialist nearly two years later. This specialist ruled no biopsy was necessary. He again appealed – this time, successfully. Unfortunately, it was too late. The blemishes were cancerous, and Laird had to have half of his nose removed.

–Coburn Report [9]

Even though we always had dozens of veterans waiting for heart surgery, Mark frequently and ironically lamented that we weren't filling up our allotted operating room "block time." He worried that the OR scheduling committee would take away the valuable OR time that was reserved for our service if it was "underutilized." And he would often confide to me his fears that other VA hospitals in our administrative region, or "VISN," would persuade Washington to shut down the cardiac surgery program at our VA, thereby reducing competition for themselves and more securely justifying their own existence.

Before any given service meeting would wrap up, I would also offer a few words about each of the patients on the general thoracic waiting list. In some ways, our problems on the thoracic side of things were the opposite of those on cardiac: too many patients who were ready to go to the OR, and only three OR slots *per month* to provide general thoracic surgery. If a patient showed up with a new lung cancer, even with a carefully completed assessment of disease stage and in good shape for curative surgery, it could be six weeks or more before the next available open slot.

I felt a particular responsibility toward the patients waiting for surgery on the general thoracic list and spent extra time with Dallis outside

---

[9] pp. 23–4.

of our service meetings each week looking for ways to jumpstart the system. Somehow we muddled through and rearranged schedules whenever we could. Sometimes we cannibalized cardiac OR time and substituted a thoracic patient, which not only helped the cancer patients, but also helped Mark keep precious cardiothoracic OR block time from going unutilized.

All in all, we tried hard to keep up with the referrals, and we tried to keep the level of modern oncology care up to the standards practiced for private patients at the university. But there was always resistance; there were always obstacles . . .

Over the years, I continued to ask Michael Baker about our ill-fated quest to obtain acceptable mediastinoscopy equipment. The conversation itself became a bit of an unconsecrated ritual. As time passed, our dialogue about the equipment was transformed further into a kind of reality check, a secret exchange of sorts that confirmed for each of us that the other understood exactly what type of bureaucracy we were a part of, exactly what we were up against in our desire to do good and to maintain our sanity at the same time. We were both committed to our patients, and deep down we both knew that one day there might be a patient who would really need up-to-date mediastinoscopy equipment to have the best chance of survival. But that imperative gradually paled against the more formidable recognition of a system that resisted change.

"So, have you contacted the vendors they use over at UCSF?" I might choose to ask one day.

"They're not on our approved vendors list, but I've got a call into one of the reps to see if they can suggest another place where we can look."

"You know, I worry that the stuff we're using is going to fall apart one day inside someone's chest—just when the bleeding starts."

"I know, Dr. Mann. I know. Most of it's already falling apart just sitting on the nurse's table."

Eventually, long before any real hope of replacing the mediastinoscopy equipment materialized, Michael achieved the promotion he was really after and was put in charge of the cardiac operating room. Cardiac surgery, even at the San Francisco VA, still had a mystique about it, and it still required an even more specialized and meticulous set of skills than other operative specialties. The cardiac room also saw complex surgeries four days a week—at least on weeks without cancellations—compared to the three days per month we were given to treat lung cancer and other general thoracic problems. Michael had worked hard to earn that promotion. He had done a very commendable job for us in the thoracic room in the absence of any real support or any established precedent, and he had helped us get a wider array of cases done than had been attempted at the San Francisco facility for years.

"Just remember, Dr. Mann," Michael would always tell me at the end of one of our discussions of the Holy Grail of updated mediastinoscopy equipment, "this is still the VA."

CHAPTER FIVE

Better than Nothing?

The VA motto was taken from Abraham Lincoln's second inaugural address in 1865: "To care for him who bore the battle and for his widow, and his orphan." Moving words. Unfortunately, by the late twentieth and early twenty-first centuries, "Something is better than nothing" might have been a more appropriate summation of the VA. Nothing reflected the mediocrity of the VA better than the experiences of vets themselves.

- *Mr. Wollenz*

One late night during my early days as an attending, I had been in the intensive care unit at the San Francisco VA assisting the residents in the care of a critically ill patient. In a quiet moment, I decided to visit another of my patients, Mr. Joseph Wollenz, who had also had a bit of a stormy post-op course and had been transferred out of the ICU earlier in the day.

Like many patients who come into surgery in frail health—and many patients at the VA in particular—Mr. Wollenz's post-op course had been complicated by "mental status changes": delirium, disorientation, and apparent hallucinations. Having scanned his brain to rule out stroke, and having tested his blood for other "metabolic" causes, this problem was ascribed to "ICU psychosis." A real medical phenomenon, but one that was "diagnosed" in this way by ruling out other specific causes of brain dysfunction, ICU psychosis was a severe disorientation that can accompany even a modestly prolonged stay in intensive care. In the ICU, day-night cycles are disrupted by constant activity, unfamiliar faces often come and go in rapid succession, and there are intense shifts between pain and drug-induced narcosis. Although the resulting "psychosis" is often treated initially with further pharmacologic disruption of brain function at the hands of psychotropic drugs, the definitive treatment for ICU psychosis is childishly simple: remove the patient from the ICU.

Since all parameters indicated that Mr. Wollenz had recovered adequately enough from his operation physiologically to be transferred to the "step-down unit," we had decided earlier that day to move him away from the one-to-one care (and behavior management) of the ICU. And since his erratic behavior would not immediately resolve, we knew that he would need a "sitter," a nursing assistant who would remain in his room and make sure he did not do anything that might be dangerous to himself or to others.

Given the tenuousness of Mr. Wollenz's condition, I had decided to head over to his ward during a quiet moment in the ICU.

Sleep deprivation is one of the most disruptive aspects of hospitalization; normal mental functioning becomes close to impossible. It is therefore essential that a hospital staff strives to provide a calm, quiet environment to promote good "sleep hygiene," often supplemented by the mildest possible sleep-inducing drugs.

For a patient, restful sleep is a blessing, but the patient's rest is not necessarily a blessing for a sitter. On overnight shifts especially, a sitter can have one of the most tedious jobs in the hospital. Sitters are therefore often desperate to keep themselves occupied. Because sitters had been assigned to many of my previous VA patients, I was not at all surprised to hear a television blaring loudly inside Mr. Wollenz's room as I approached down the corridor of Ward 3B.

As was my habit, I knocked on Mr. Wollenz's door before I entered. There was no response. And when I tried to push the door open, I met resistance. Assuming that hospital paraphernalia like a bedside tray stand had migrated and was blocking the door, I knocked again, this time more loudly, with the expectation that the sitter would let me in. When there was again no response, I called out, again with no results.

Deeply puzzled, I walked to the nursing station just a few feet away from Mr. Wollenz's room. This was by intention; we wanted nurses close by. I was not surprised, however, to find that no one at all was there—typical for a nursing station at the VA at night. So I headed toward an area where I knew the nurses often congregated for breaks.

And, true to form, I found three nurses there, sitting comfortably, chatting over coffee, somewhat startled by my abrupt entrance. "I can't get into Mr. Wollenz's room," I announced. "Where is his sitter?"

"Oh, she had to go home, and we couldn't find anybody else."

"What? Why weren't we notified?"

"Oh, I'm pretty sure we tried calling the resident, but he didn't answer. Anyway, the patient's been very quiet."

"Well, there seems to be something stuck in front of his door. Can someone help me get inside?"

After several glances back and forth among the three nurses, one reluctantly inched his way up out of his chair and followed me slowly back toward Mr. Wollenz's room. I demonstrated that the door only moved a few inches from the doorpost, and the nurse, with an air of disdain and exuding a sense of problem-solving capability, thrust his weight against the door with all his might.

"Ohhh!" The groan was almost bone chilling, emanating from behind the door that remained mostly closed, although it had swung open another foot with the force of the nurse's body. The eerie glow of the television in the otherwise darkened room simply added to the surreal nature of the unfolding scene. As the nurse and I looked down and could now see around the edge of the door, it was quite apparent that it was, in fact, Mr. Wollenz himself who had been acting as a doorstop.

Through the small opening in the doorway, a distinct stench was also better able to seep out from within the darkened room. The groan had elicited an instinctive recoil from the nurse, which relieved some of the added pressure and discomfort on the incapacitated patient. The two of us slipped through the crack in the door and knelt down beside the crumpled Mr. Wollenz. He was lying in a pool of his own urine and feces. He was conscious and able to follow simple commands, though he was only minimally responsive. I quickly assessed for evidence of a fractured spine, and after satisfying myself that there was little danger in moving this huddled mass of humanity, we lifted the patient off the soiled floor and back into his empty bed.

It became apparent through questioning that it had been several hours since the sitter had announced her needed departure. Although no authorization had been obtained from a responsible physician, the nurses had determined on their own that the proximity of Mr. Wollenz's room to the nurse's station obviated any real need for a sitter inside his room. It wasn't long before Mr. Wollenz and his special needs had been forgotten, and the nurses' duties and desire for a coffee and chat drew all of them away from the ward's main nursing desk. At some point during the one-and-a-half to two hours before my arrival, when the nursing station was essentially abandoned, Mr. Wollenz had become confused enough to pull himself out of bed and wander toward the door, which had been left ajar to aid in the nurse's surveillance (they had not, however, thought to shut off the television, which had likely precluded any real chance for the man to sleep). Perhaps Mr. Wollenz had even been lucid enough to know he needed to go to the bathroom; in any event, his unwitnessed collapse threw his body against the door, shutting out any hope of further monitoring and relegating him to lie in his own waste until I had happened by.

Eventually, Mr. Wollenz regained most, but not all, of his preoperative mental capacity and was discharged to a local rehabilitation facility. Although I spoke with the ward's charge nurse the next morning, there was no follow-up on why our order for a twenty-four-hour sitter had essentially been discarded as inconvenient and unnecessary, nor were there any repercussions for the nurses who had been on duty that night. It had not been the first time that such an order would go unfilled, nor certainly the last.

> In court filings detailing the V.A. response to other problems, Dr. Ram Chaturvedi, formerly with the Dallas V.A. Medical Center, said that he began complaining in 2008 about shoddy patient care, including negligence by nurses who had marked the wrong kidney while preparing a patient for a procedure. In another

instance, Dr. Chaturvedi said medical personnel had brought the wrong patient to an operating table. A supervisor told Dr. Chaturvedi to "let some things slide" because of staffing problems, but he continued writing up complaints. Officials considered him disruptive and fired him in 2010.

—The New York Times [10]

• *Mr. Moran*

Sometimes our inability to give the vets what they deserved had nothing to do with the will, the enthusiasm, or the confidence of the practitioners. Take, for example, the case of Greg Moran. Interestingly, Mr. Moran did not consider himself a lucky person to begin with. As evidence, he'd point out that he had tried and failed to avoid the draft, and he had tried and failed to stay out of combat in Southeast Asia. But he returned alive and intact, and later ascribed that to the bad luck of remaining without any significant service-connected disability. Still he valued being able to come to the VA to get his healthcare and particularly his medications. Although abstinent at the time, he had battled alcoholism for much of his life. The addiction had certainly taken its toll; he had married, had children, and had divorced within just a few years of returning from military service. Although his children and he lived in the same area and knew how to contact each other, they rarely saw each other more than once per decade.

Greg Moran had probably had a bout with rheumatic fever at some point during his hard life. Likely caused by an untreated infection of his throat with a common bacterium, the disease led to scarring and thickening of the leaflets of his heart's aortic valve. Although his heart had been able to compensate for the added stress of pumping against a sticky valve, the strain of overload would continue to take its toll, and surgical

---

[10] Eric Lichtblau, "V.A. Punished Critics on Staff, Doctors Assert," *The New York Times*, June 15, 2014, accessed June 17, 2014, http://www.nytimes.com/2014/06/16/us/va-punished-critics-on-staff-doctors-assert.html.

replacement of the valve was felt by surgeons at the San Francisco VA to be the best way to prevent eventual heart failure and a cardiac death.

Like many previous alcoholics, Mr. Moran's teeth were not in the best shape. Although salvageable, he would need some time to clean up multiple infections of his teeth and gums. It was essential that his mouth be as free of infection as possible prior to implanting an artificial heart valve that would itself be highly susceptible to infection. His heart operation was not a true emergency, but the cardiac surgeons at the San Francisco VA were under pressure to utilize their OR time, and Mr. Moran was the only patient otherwise ready for surgery that week. Told that he required urgent intervention, he was brought first to the oral surgery suite for extraction of all of his teeth, the fastest way possible to clear the infection of his mouth. The next day, he was brought to the operating room for aortic valve replacement.

The replacement of Mr. Moran's valve went smoothly, and he recovered well from surgery. But as the early days after his operation rolled by and he was transferred from the ICU onto our regular postoperative ward, Mr. Moran was stunned to learn that, having suddenly lost all of his teeth, the VA did not provide any benefits for dentures.

Mr. Moran was assigned the task of nourishing his healing chest and heart on a diet of liquids and pureed foods, with a wish of good luck at finding some way to finance a new set of teeth. Dallis attempted to console the man, but consolation for him was a thin meal.

One might have thought that the lack of foresight and planning for Mr. Moran's dental recovery might have spawned a concerted effort to address this programmatic flaw. It did not. In fact, the problem with Mr. Moran's problem was that he was neither the first nor the last veteran to wind up with a shiny new heart valve—and toothless. Even Dallis became resigned to having that difficult conversation, explaining to the aching, post-op patient that, no, the VA, having removed all of his teeth, was not going to replace them. Even for Dallis, as relentless as she was in overcoming the system, that part of the system was just another unfortunate reality for the vets.

- *Mr. Carney*

Another unfortunate reality was that, no matter which VA hospital you might be talking about, things often just did not get done. Dan Carney was a cheerfully garrulous veteran of the Korean War whom I met on a rotation at the Palo Alto VA Hospital during my general surgery residency. He was a diabetic with nonhealing ulcers on his feet caused by poor circulation. Ulcers that might have been prevented with special "orthotic" shoes designed precisely for people prone to this type of injury.

Mr. Carney had indomitably high spirits. By the time we met, he was about to have his left foot cut off to prevent a potentially lethal spread of infection up his leg and into his bloodstream. He had already been held captive in the hospital for weeks by my predecessors on the service, receiving an escalating variety of intravenous antibiotics intended to stem the progress of infection marching up his foot and leg. Unfortunately, they had not.

Mr. Carney often joked during his ordeal, but he seemed to laugh most about his custom-made orthotic shoes. Despite a long history of ulcers, and despite the fact that he routinely sought care at the VA for years, no one had thought to intervene early, when the simple solution of an appropriate shoe might have made all the difference to his imperiled left foot.

Instead, Mr. Carney's non-orthotic shoes inevitably continued to engender ulcers that threatened not to heal. I learned from my frequent, long conversations with the loquacious vet that, without his own means of transportation and without easy access to the few VA shuttles, it was not easy for Mr. Carney to keep his appointments at vascular wound clinics. Rather than recognize this obvious pattern and find an alternative means of providing either better transportation or better patient education and self-care training (together with appropriate home nursing visits), the VA chose simply to keep rescheduling his missed appointments, often without making sure the patient knew when he was next expected to appear. Ulcers that might have healed with true, early "aggressive local wound care" instead festered under bandages that sometimes lingered on his feet for months. These did nothing to prevent the advent of gangrene. Now, his leg—and potentially his life—was threatened by infection, and he would soon undergo amputation below the knee.

The irresistible joke to Mr. Carney, however, and one that he laughed at without a trace of bitterness, was that while his foot continued to rot quite unattractively in his hospital bed, a black left orthosis still sat shiny and new in its box back at his home. By the time the shoe had been prescribed and made, he would tell us with a wink, his gangrenous foot required too much bandaging for him to be able to wear the specially fitted device. In the end, it seemed even funnier to poor Mr. Carney that with the final solution of amputation, necessitated by VA treatment that had been simply too little, too late, the shoe would never have a chance to sit around the one foot for which it had been expressly created.

During my tenure on the vascular service at the Palo Alto VA Hospital, the large majority of amputees had lost their feet or legs years—often decades—after returning home from military service. They had not been injured by grenades or hidden explosives. Instead, they were the victims of diabetes and vascular disease, often underdiagnosed and undertreated. Their limbs had been ravaged from the inside, often by an insidious lack of oxygen due to poor circulation. The injuries that eventually led to loss of limb in these former soldiers were almost never inflicted by shrapnel. Instead they arose from circumstances as innocuous as an abrasion from ill-fitting shoes, or by stepping on broken glass with a foot rendered insensate by long-standing diabetes.

> Veteran Larry Wilkinson of Colorado said his doctor never called him with test results after he sought treatment at a VA medical center for a foot infection. Mr. Wilkinson had to have his leg amputated when he still had not heard from his doctor after two months. In describing his experience, he aptly stated, "I feel the VA owes me a leg."
>
> –Coburn Report [11]

---

[11] p. 24.

* * *

In recent decades, VA mediocrities have not gone completely unnoticed. In fact, by 1986, Congress had gotten very upset about the very low level of care that was being documented at VA facilities around the country. Showing unusual resolve, Congress enacted legislation aimed at improving the veterans' care. Realizing that the institution's back might be up against a wall, VA leadership instituted a number of programs in response to that legislation that eventually led to a self-proclaimed "transformation" of the VA into a provider of superlative health care by the late 1990s.

One remedial VA program was the National Surgery Quality Improvement Program. Like many federal and military-related programs, it became known by its acronym, NSQIP, pronounced "nisskwip." As Mark Ratcliffe first explained it to me in 2004 or 2005, NSQIP—or more specifically the VA programs that eventually spawned NSQIP—were initially conceived to fulfill a specific congressional mandate for improvement in the veterans' surgical outcomes. But the VA leadership had apparently taken that congressional cue and had run with the ball far beyond anyone's wildest expectations.

NSQIP was all about the data. In fact, by 2005, the VA was routinely collecting an enormous set of data on every patient undergoing surgery at VA hospitals, adding up to hundreds of thousands of operations. At the end of each year, they would analyze the year's mountain of data to identify preoperative "risk factors" that could assess which patients had been more likely to do worse. The VA's annual "statistical model" then allowed administrators to assess how many deaths or complications should have occurred at any given hospital based both on nationwide VA averages and on the unique makeup of each hospital's actual patient population. Such a statistical system was revolutionary. Hospitals that had experienced significantly fewer surgical deaths than expected were praised as "low outliers." Of course, there were "high outliers," as well.

But there was an even more important, and unexpected, outcome of NSQIP: the VA discovered that simply by telling each hospital how it was doing, by telling the best hospitals that they had the best surgical records and the worst hospitals that they were the worst, surgical outcomes began steadily improving throughout the VA system. Not just at the weaker institutions, but everywhere.

Although impressed by the magnitude and rigor of NSQIP, when I first learned of the dramatic, system-wide improvements in outcomes, I found them a little hard to believe. The improvements were noticed before any comprehensive system had been put into place for the weaker facilities to benefit from the experience of their stronger counterparts. Apparently not wanting to rock a successful boat, the VA never pushed for such a system to materialize. Even more confusing, there wasn't any bona-fide scientific explanation for the substantial improvements seen even at the average and above-average facilities. Skeptical as I might have been in 2005, little did I suspect then the potentially devastating effect that NSQIP could have on individual patients.

Mark Ratcliffe, on the other hand, had a profound enthusiasm for NSQIP. The San Francisco VA, he was eager to point out in 2005, had been the only VA hospital to be a "low outlier" in six of the seven years since the success of NSQIP had first been published. That meant that compared to the VA average across the system, only the San Francisco VA had consistently, year in and year out, observed significantly fewer surgical deaths than this revolutionary statistical model would have predicted.

By 2005, NSQIP had already been proven to be a remarkable success. Based entirely on the VA's NSQIP experience, the American College of Surgeons, the leading academic organization for surgeons nationally, had already begun to test an application of the system in American hospitals outside of the VA. Dutiful, inquisitive academics that we were, Mark and I began to wonder why this type of remarkable, unprecedented improvement in care needed to be limited to surgery alone. If NSQIP had uncovered a previously unsuspected method to improve healthcare, shouldn't the practice of internal medicine benefit from such a discovery, as well?

Bolstered by a sense of quality improvement genius coming off our own local NSQIP success, we proposed to our influential California Senator—and San Francisco native—Diane Feinstein that she sponsor a sister VA program that would expand NSQIP in this new direction. Not wanting to stray too far from the NSQIP example, we switched out the word "surgical" for "medical," and simply termed our brainchild

"NMQIP." Of course, we also proposed, given its NSQIP prowess, that the San Francisco VA ought to carry the banner and lead a pilot NMQIP development program. To our great surprise, the senator followed through on our suggestion, and a NMQIP-style proposal made it into a legislative initiative introduced by her later that year. To no one's great surprise, however, the legislation never made it to the president's desk.

CHAPTER SIX

Being There

Slowly, I began to accept that trying to improve things at the San Francisco VA was like trying to run through a pool of molasses. Despite the "transformation" of the 1990s, there were obstacles, great and small, that just seemed to crop up everywhere you would turn. Obstacles that just didn't need to be there. Often little things that made it more difficult to get anything done. Things that made one wonder if anyone was thinking about the reason why the institution existed in the first place.

It may seem to be a trivial issue, but when physicians need to divide their time between urban hospitals, they need to have quick transportation back and forth. There are numerous unforeseeable demands often pulling them in opposite directions. And so most hospitals make arrangements for clinicians to be able to drive up and deposit their cars somewhere safe and out of the way. Not the San Francisco VA. I regularly needed to run from clinical or educational activities at UCSF and head straight to the San Francisco VA, either for an outpatient clinic or even for an operation. Whether or not a patient was waiting to go under anesthesia, and no matter if twenty patients were lining up in clinic, I would need to drive around for twenty or thirty minutes, desperately seeking a parking space either on campus or in the busy neighborhood outside.

Interspersed around the buildings of the San Francisco VA campus, there were hundreds of parking spaces. With such a modest volume of healthcare in our 150-bed facility, it amazed me that those hundreds of parking spaces would fill up every morning well before nine o'clock. As I drove around and around, I would wonder where in the world all these people who had successfully parked all these cars actually worked. What did they all do? They couldn't all be caring for the handful of inpatients, nor could they be flooding our understaffed clinics. There were, on the other hand, many corridors of administrative offices and many other non-clinical places for these people to be working. And to be contributing to that that sixty-plus billion dollar budget.

One morning, after my usual thirty minutes of driving up and down the back alleys and dirt paths of the San Francisco VA, and even after cruising the surrounding neighborhood for a place to park, I left the car in a spot near one of the main VA buildings that was clearly marked: "For Authorized Government Vehicles Only." I felt that I had little choice; patients had already been waiting an inordinate amount of time in my clinic and further delay seemed unconscionable. I stopped by the San Francisco VA Security Office on my way into the clinic, which had a service window that was staffed by a female member of the San Francisco VA police force at the time.

"Hi!" I said to the officer, trying to be as cheerful and as encouraging of a collaborative attitude as possible. "I'm Dr. Mann." As I spoke, I pointed to the red embroidery on my long, white coat. "I just want to let you guys know that there was absolutely no place to park this morning. I'm already very late for a busy clinic, so I parked my car in one of the spots reserved for government vehicles near the cafeteria."

"Yeah," the utterly uninterested policewoman responded, "so what do you want me to do about it?"

"It would be great if you could let whoever needs to know not to give the car a ticket and not to tow it, and that I'll move it right after clinic."

"Sorry, we can't do that. And besides, you're not allowed to park there."

It was at moments like these that the patience that had been forged over the course of ten years of residency really came in handy.

"Yes, I realize that the space is supposed to be off limits, but I think it's pretty clear that these are extenuating circumstances since there are patients waiting to be seen and treated."

"We can't make any allowances for any extenuating circumstances, so you'll have to go and move your car."

"Actually," collaboration was not working, and so I switched gears into a more aggressive stance, "I happen to know that this problem was brought to the attention of the chief of staff recently. My service chief told me that doctors are now authorized to park anywhere if the parking shortage may impact patient care."

This was true, at least to some degree, though I had my doubts that any official edicts had been passed down, or that anyone in the police force was really ready to give any of the physicians a break.

"We haven't been told about any changes to the parking policy. I can give you my supervisor's email address and you can ask him about it yourself. But he's not on campus right now, so unless you want a ticket, you had better move your car."

Even a decade of residency allows one to build up only so much patience.

"Officer, look, this is a hospital. We're not here to administer pensions or monitor the progress of highway construction. We're here to treat patients—veterans—many of whom have life-threatening illnesses." The indifference on the woman's face was palpable and imposing, but I carried on. "These men are sick and tired, and they're also sick and tired of waiting for me to show up, so there's no way I'm going to spend another minute driving my car in search of a parking spot that doesn't exist."

"Well then, you'll probably get a ticket and maybe towed."

At this point, I was willing to cut my losses and chose a different tactic of negotiation entirely.

"All right, then, can you at least notify someone so they don't tow the damn car?"

"Sorry, we don't handle the towing, and I don't got no way to notify no one."

The proliferating negatives made it clear that this conversation had been about as fruitful as my initial search for a parking spot. Imagining the increasingly anxious looks on the faces of my patients and my clinic staff, I turned and began a defeated retreat toward the clinic. Not satisfied with her simple victory, the VA policewoman suddenly displayed a burst of uncharacteristic vitality and called out, "Doctor, one second please."

I turned around, foolishly hoping that I had inspired either a kernel of common sense or at least some sympathy for my patients.

"It looks like you're wearing scrubs under that white coat. If you've just gotten here, that means that you were wearing VA scrubs outside of VA property. We've instituted a new policy and we're cracking down on people who leave the premises with our scrubs, so I gotta warn you that if we see you going or coming wearing VA property again, you're going to be cited and arrested."

＊ ＊ ＊

One week, Dallis was uncharacteristically late for one of our hour-long thoracic planning sessions—the one hour per week she allotted to manage the long list of patients waiting for thoracic surgery. She was clearly exasperated and dejected, and I asked her what was wrong.

"What's wrong? Really? You want to know what's wrong? Okay, I'll tell you what's wrong. I've just been arguing with a brain-dead clerk in the transportation office, that's what's wrong. Any other questions, Dr. Mann?"

Her anger and exasperation were hardly rare, but every time one of our patients needed a special consideration after surgery, Dallis somehow managed to block out her past experience of the institution and suspend her disbelief that positive change was possible.

"Dare I ask what it was about?"

Dallis didn't really need my prompting; she was eager to blow off steam. She had simply been allowing her engines to cool down a bit so she could catch her breath and get the story off her chest.

"Mr. Johnson needs a way to get home, and I'm running into walls trying to get him there." Mr. Johnson had had lung cancer surgery about a week earlier.

"Physical Therapy finally signed off on him," she continued, "and so he's cleared to go home today. But he lives in Richmond [a town in the East Bay, across the Bay Bridge from San Francisco, many miles away from the VA campus], and there's nobody who can come pick him up. So I went to the Transportation Office to make an arrangement for him, and they told me he didn't qualify. He lives too close, and he's not service connected enough or some such thing."

"And so they want him to walk home?"

"Well, I suggested at least a taxi voucher."

"A taxi?" That did not strike me as a good idea. Although the Physical Therapy Department had evaluated his condition and his needs at home, his ability to get himself out of bed, his ability to climb steps, and so on, there is a reason why newly discharged hospital patients are traditionally pushed in wheel chairs to a waiting family's arms and opened car doors. Mr. Johnson was still severely weakened and in significant pain after we had opened up his rib cage. In fact, we had pulled it apart with heavy steel retractors during the couple of hours it took us to dig a life-threatening tumor out of his lung. The simple act of coughing was extremely painful to him; he could not reasonably have been expected to lug his belongings home himself. During the inevitable jostling of a journey home, he was likely to experience an array of troubling symptoms ranging from increased pain to severe nausea or lightheadedness. It made little sense to ask a taxi driver to take responsibility for a patient on what could be more than an hour-long journey across San Francisco Bay.

"Do you really think it's appropriate," I ventured gingerly, hoping not to upset the tinderbox that was still Dallis's nerves, "to send Mr. Johnson home in a taxi?"

"No, and neither does the Transportation Office."

Well, that was surprising, but also reassuring. Despite what must have been a mountain of regulations, the folks in this administrative office were able to see through the protocols, and had actually understood a veteran's difficult situation and had acted with compassion.

"They're sending him home on a bus and the subway instead."

If Dallis Manwaring and Marc Marcotte were two shining beacons floating on the sometimes dismal and disquieting sea of clinical medicine at the San Francisco VA, there were also a few bright spots on the administrative side, as well. A group of longtime VA staffers sat at desks that occupied a central workspace in the Surgical Service's suite of offices. One of them was Nakia Branner. She was a tall African

American woman in her thirties, level headed, calm, and very polite. She knew very well why she was there at the VA: to push papers. But she had a keen understanding of how meaningful that paper pushing could actually be. She knew that she was supporting surgeons. Surgeons who were, to the best of their ability, making differences in veterans' lives every day. And she knew that without the stream of paper that she kept flowing, everything would come to a grinding halt. She had been at the VA for a long time, long enough to know exactly how to keep things flowing. And she did.

It was Nakia who explained to me one day a key element of our monthly Surgical Service meetings. These were meetings that were convened in the San Francisco VA's largest auditorium one Tuesday morning each month. The entire cadre of full-time and part-time surgeons was supposed to attend these monthly meetings. Good luck. It was unrealistic to expect such a varied group of extremely busy academic surgeons with numerous other responsibilities related to patient care, education, and research—all at multiple venues—to set aside the same time slot on their calendars. But there were numerous emails about the need not just to attend Surgical Service meetings, but to attend them *on time*. One trick busy surgeons often used to get more done than is humanly possible was to show up late. The emails seemed to indicate that that was not going to be an option. Nakia, in her unmistakably kind and gentle voice, was happy to help me understand why.

"Dr. Ratcliffe really wants everybody to start attending these meetings, Dr. Mann," Nakia started off, taking things slow. "He's going to have someone taking attendance, so you're gonna have to sign in and someone's gonna have to make sure that it was really you."

Nakia paused slightly, making sure that I was still with her.

"The sign-in sheet used to be on the outside of the auditorium, but they moved it inside, and someone's going to be right there watching everybody sign in. I think they usually lock the doors when the meeting starts, so if you don't get there on time, you won't be able to sign the sheet."

As Nakia paused again, a slightly devilish look was very slowly, almost imperceptibly, marching across her face.

"This is the VA, Dr. Mann. All you got to worry about is checking the boxes. That's all they care about, you know. They've just got to see that the boxes were checked. And you know, they always care most about certain boxes. So if you make sure to know which ones are the most important, and then you make sure to check those boxes, you'll end up being just fine. It doesn't matter what you actually do, so long as you checked the right box.

"Dr. Ratcliffe really wants people to attend these meetings," she continued, making sure I got the full benefit of her admonition. "He wants everybody's signature on that sign-in sheet. They're going to be paying a lot of attention to who checked that box. But once you're signed in, they don't care at all what you actually do. You can just sit down and go to sleep, you know, rest a little bit 'cause it'll be so early and everything. There'll be lots of people sleeping at that meeting and no one cares at all. As long as you signed in, as long as you checked the box."

I was struck by the stark clarity of Nakia's insight. It would be years before I could appreciate the full depth and breadth of what Nakia had perceived and had articulated so clearly. Whether it had taken her years, or whether her high EQ had allowed her to home in much more quickly than I on the reality of the VA enterprise, I would never know. But I remained grateful to Nakia for accelerating my learning curve in this respect. Neither this nor any other pieces of her advice ever led me astray.

Nakia helped me to understand that success at the VA was mostly about being there.

* * *

And then there was Terry Kerry-Gourneau. If Nakia was an inherently peaceful and quiet woman, Terry was on the other end of the spectrum. Boisterous and always full of good cheer, Terry sat opposite Nakia in the surgical suite, her desk situated strategically against a wall shared by my own office. She was middle aged, and though she certainly had her own share of personal challenges to overcome, she always seemed quite strong and robust. She was always able to look on the bright side, and she often regaled us with stories of being out and about with her small, precious dog.

Terry was my timekeeper. Why did I need a timekeeper? In an admission of the type of medical practitioner the VA seemed to realize they were able to attract, the institution had developed a deep-seated mistrust of its part-time physician staff. They must have discovered decades of accounting abuse and embezzlement of pay for shifts that were never worked. And so an elaborate system had evolved to keep on eye on the rogue physicians. Part-time doctors were paid for hours they spent at the VA, according to a "tour of duty" to which they were assigned. That tour dictated which hours on which day of the week the physician needed to be present. These hours were tracked, and a timekeeper was necessary to keep a watchful eye on the veracity of the tracking. Beyond a simple timekeeper, there were audits and surprise visits by third-party examiners, who would come searching for physicians during hours and the locations prescribed by their tours.

As Nakia taught me, it was all about checking the box. The VA desperately wanted to know that it hadn't been duped into paying someone for an hour during which they might have been somewhere else. The VA cared nothing about what the doctor actually did. No accountability for seeing patients or for their outcomes. In fact there was no other yardstick beyond just being there. To be fair, this system might have made a little more sense for part-time physicians from private practice who came to the VA for specific clinics or even for specific blocks of operating room time. But it made no sense whatsoever for the very numerous part-time physicians who, like me, were academics from the medical schools with which the VA famously had developed such close ties. We were not paid by the VA to sit in a chair; the VA paid us to make sure the vets were being cared for, to make sure the residents were being supervised and taught, to make sure clinical programs did not fall apart, and to do groundbreaking research.

None of that could be boiled to a set of hours that would be the same week in and week out. Nor did it ever happen in the same particular places each week. On the other hand, it would have been completely obvious to tell whether or not we were doing the jobs for which we were really getting paid—all one had to do was to look at the results. In fact, if an academic was working the same hours each week, that was a pretty clear sign that he or she probably wasn't doing his or her job, at least not doing it very well.

But these time and attendance boxes were clearly boxes that the VA needed to have checked—big time. Our hospital administrators quaked in their boots at the thought of a time and attendance auditor who showed up and had trouble finding any particular doctor during his tour of duty. And so the timekeepers had the additionally painful job of making sure the professors had at least let them know where they would be during the tour, and if possible indicate in an official note ahead of time that they were going to be doing something reasonable somewhere else.

> The Department [of Veteran Affairs] has long delayed developing a standard methodology to measure physician productivity, a practice standard in private-sector programs and Medicare. Government auditors first made the recommendation to establish this type of standard in 1981. Since then, the auditors [Government Accounting Office and the Inspector General] have issued another six reports with essentially the same recommendation. Yet, by late 2013, the VA had still not developed an adequate and comprehensive means of measuring physician productivity and determining staffing needs. . . . VA physicians take far fewer patients than a typical doctor in the private sector. An average private-sector primary care physician has an average caseload of 2,300, according to a study in the *Annals of Family Medicine*. Yet, the VA targets panel sizes of 1,200 for its physicians - almost half the workload of private-sector providers.
>
> –Coburn Report [12]

In addition to all of her other administrative responsibilities, including being the administrative assistant to Mark Ratcliffe, Terry was my timekeeper. She cheerfully tried to keep up with my hectic

---

[12] p. 27.

work. But what I valued most was her irrepressible good spirits, even in the face of a bureaucracy she knew often kept her from making reasonable decisions about how to do even the more reasonable parts of her job. Sure, it didn't hurt that every time I walked through the office, she would shout out, "Hey, Dr. Mann, did you know you're our favorite?!" She may have had other favorites; I never asked. But my attitude seemed different enough from the run-of-the-mill participant in the VA machinery that I at least kidded myself into thinking that the title might reasonably have been mine.

Back in the OR, there was Michael Baker. He, too, seemed to recognize that we were trying to do something special at the San Francisco VA, something that the vets particularly deserved. One day, we were preparing for surgery to remove from a patient a very dangerous lung cancer. The odds were tough in this case, both because the cancer may have already spread to lymph nodes in the patient's chest and because the depth of the tumor in his lung might require us to remove not just the one cancerous section, or "lobe," but the entire lung itself. If the cancer had spread, the patient's chances to be cured of this often fatal disease would be drastically reduced; and if we had to remove his entire lung, his chance of having complications or even of dying because of the operation would seriously increase.

To address the first issue of tumor spread, we would begin the complex procedure with a smaller, preliminary mediastinoscopy. That "minor" procedure would involve a three-centimeter incision at the base of the patient's neck and would allow us to explore the middle of his chest through a deep, narrow, and dark hole. To address the second issue, the entire operative team would need to be on top of its game; we would have to dissect down to the root of the lung, where enormous blood vessels carried half of the blood that would be pumped out of the heart with each beat. We would then pick our way meticulously through tough scar tissue and rocklike calcifications and peel the tumor very carefully away from normal lung.

"Dr. Mann?" The slight twang of Michael Baker's voice was unmistakable; his tone was typically cheerful but matter-of-fact. "Can I talk with you for just a minute?"

Since Michael was the nurse in charge of the thoracic OR, I was expecting a review of critical details essential to adequately prepare for what was going to be an extremely difficult case.

I was wrong.

"Say, listen, Dr. Mann," he began as soon as the two of us had migrated to a quiet corner of the large operating room, "you must have heard gossip around this place. It goes on all the time." I gave him a nod. I had. VAs, in general, tended to be bubbling cauldrons of gossip; there was even more of it there than I'd experienced at other, non-VA hospitals. But I made every effort I could to avoid it. I wanted to stay as far as possible from that kind of poisonous chatter.

"I hate the way people gossip around this place," Michael pressed on. "I mean, it gets in the way of our doing our jobs. As if it weren't hard enough for us to get things done around here in the first place."

"Yes," I replied, trying to find a way to be supportive while deflecting what I feared was an attempt to draw me into the very gossip he was deploring. "I know exactly what you mean," I replied neutrally, "and I appreciate that you make an effort not to get involved."

"Well, thanks, Dr. Mann." He seemed genuinely flattered, but at the same time undeterred. "Some of the stuff you hear out in the OR lounge is just stupid," he pressed further, "but I worry that some of it could be dangerous."

Now Michael had gotten my attention, and I decided to hear him out.

"I don't know where they come up with some of this stuff, but I thought I should warn you that I overheard a couple of people talking about you as I was getting ready for the case. I couldn't hear what they were saying, but it didn't exactly sound like they were singing your praises."

The cryptic nature of Michael's words was made all the more mysterious by his unperturbed affect. Confused but intrigued, I simply asked him what he thought he had heard.

"I really couldn't say for sure, Dr. Mann, but I think you're a better thoracic surgeon than we've had out here in years, and I've really enjoyed working with you. You really care an awful lot about your patients. Plus

I think you're a really nice guy. So I just wanted to make sure you knew to watch your back a little more out here than you're probably used to doing over at UC. I just wanted to make sure you knew that people had a way of getting back at folks out here that you might not be used to."

"Getting back?" I asked instinctively, "At me? For what? Is there something I've done that's gotten people upset?"

Michael Baker's eyes smiled above his surgical facemask.

"C'mon, Dr. Mann, you know you've pushed us to work harder out here than we're used to. That's one of the things I love about helping you in thoracic. But not everybody appreciates that. Plus, sometimes you ride us kind of hard. Not everybody out here is as clued in about what's going on in the cases as I am, and they have a hard time understanding what you're asking them to do."

"Is that what they're talking about? Is that what you've overheard?"

"No, it's other stuff, uglier stuff—nothing I want to repeat. Anyway, I don't think it's going anywhere right now, but I wanted to make sure you knew to watch your back."

That was all I was going to get out of Michael Baker. But at least he had been correct; I had truly not been aware that poisonous gossip was being used as a mechanism of retaliation. On the other hand, I wasn't entirely surprised, and it was a little reassuring to know that I had a secret ally in whatever secret war I might have fallen into. Still, this little side conversation had been disconcerting, to say the least.

"Well, thank you, Michael. I'll keep that in mind."

After a prolonged pause, I realized that there was something else I had wanted to ask.

"Say," I said cheerfully, trying to lighten up the mood of our previous conversation, "did we ever get the new mediastinoscopy set?"

Michael laughed under his mask, and shook his head in disbelief.

"You're not serious, Dr. Mann. I wrote up the order right after we talked last time, and I even showed the OR manager what our ancient setup looks like. I feel terrible every time I ask you to pick up that stuff and use it on a patient, but there's nothing more I can do. I promise I'll keep pushing, but I wouldn't hold my breath."

With a resigned shrug, I turned toward the OR door, knowing that it would still be more than an hour for my patient to get through the preparations that would have taken about twenty minutes at a private hospital. Michael was right about another important thing: the VA was not a good place to hold one's breath.

> A corrosive culture has led to personnel prob-
> lems across the Department [of Veteran Affairs]
> that are seriously impacting morale . . . a cor-
> rosive culture of distrust between some VA
> employees and management, a history of
> retaliation toward employees raising issues,
> and a lack of accountability . . . There is a cul-
> ture across much of the Department that
> encourages discontent and backlash against
> employees. Whistleblower complaints sug-
> gest poor management, and reflect a palpable
> level of frustration at the local, regional and
> National levels. As an example, approximately
> one-fourth of all whistleblower cases [the Office
> of Special Counsel] is currently reviewing
> across the Federal government come from the
> Department of Veteran Affairs.
>
> –White House Report [13]

---

[13] White House Report: "Issues Impacting Access To Timely Care At VA Medical Facilities," June 27, 2014, p. 3.

CHAPTER SEVEN

Blind Eyes Opened

"Come in and have a seat."

It was the spring of 2006, three years after my initial faculty appointment at UCSF, and once again I was meeting with our department chair, Nancy Ascher, this time for an annual career development review. Without looking up from her paperwork, Nancy beckoned me into her office. She was one of the most formidable women in American surgery, and she was my boss. Real leaders inspire respect; often they inspire awe and even anxiety. Nancy inspired all three.

As much as anything else, though, Nancy was a straight shooter. She had always seemed to respect my abilities and achievements, and we got along well. So while my visits to Nancy's office for these annual reviews were not quite relaxed and carefree, neither were they associated with any dread or trepidation.

"David tells me things are going well for you in the operating room."

At this point, Nancy had granted me her full attention. She stood up from behind her large oak desk and sat down instead in a wooden armchair, joining me at the round coffee table closer to the door of her office. Despite her positions of leadership in the medical school and the hospital, the office was still not large by corporate standards; the clutter of Nancy's many responsibilities, along with the several photos, plaques, and other mementos of an illustrious career, made the space seem smaller still.

The David whom she referenced was David Jablons, the founder of the general thoracic surgery program in our Division of Adult CT

Surgery at UCSF. By then, I had gotten to know that there was little that went on in Nancy's department that she didn't keep a watchful eye on, and she was adept at picking reliable sources of information.

"Things are going okay," I responded. There was no place for false modesty, either in the realm of surgery, with its often bombastic and narcissistic personalities, or when striving toward academic advancement. But in a place like UCSF, where renowned practitioners and researchers were common, any faculty member's success needed to be put into context.

"We're building a reputation for the aggressive management of metastatic sarcoma," I continued, filling in a little more detail than I suspected had made it into David's sound bites. "And since there aren't many sarcoma centers in this part of the country, it's resonating more and more with referring docs."

Sarcoma was a relatively rare form of cancer, and its management differed in some important ways from other malignancies that either started in or spread to the chest. So it was important for sarcoma patients to seek out expert care. In addition to operating on more garden-variety lung cancers, I had begun developing both a specialty in the treatment of sarcoma and a reputation as a thoracic surgeon who could take very difficult cases to the OR and produce good results. As a result, referrals for these kinds of challenging cases were increasingly coming to me from a widening range of outside physicians—some from competing medical centers in the Bay Area, some from as far away as Texas and Oklahoma.

This type of clinical success within her department pleased Nancy, and she did not hide her approval. But she had recruited me heavily based on my promise as a surgeon-scientist, and she had gone out on a limb promoting me among the more dedicated scientific staff who often looked down upon "dumb surgeons."

"I've also heard that you've made a few accomplishments in your research since the last time we met."

I knew immediately that the main "accomplishment" about which Nancy cared the most was the relatively recent decision by the National Institutes of Health to fund a grant application of mine known as an "R01." In biomedical research circles, approval of "peer-reviewed" funding was one of the most important benchmarks of an investigator's success. Funding from the NIH was considered an essential litmus test for any researcher who aspired not only to acceptance as a serious scientist, but who also wanted to lay claim to a leadership or groundbreaking role within his or her field. And among NIH grants, the R01 was the most coveted prize. In 2006, Draconian funding cuts had limited the approval of NIH grants to an unusually small, rarefied percentage of the best applications. *Surgeon*-scientists, with their busier schedules and often less formal scientific training compared to full-time researchers, were considered at a special disadvantage. Even in the best of times, successful faculty members achieved the granting of their first R01 an average of seven years after their initial appointment. I had gotten funding of this R01 within two and a half, and I realized at this meeting that Nancy could not only feel vindicated, but that I had given her something to brag about with her basic science colleagues.

"But what I really wanted to ask you," Nancy said after congratulating me on the R01, allowing a mischievous smile to move across her face for the first time since I had walked in the door, "is why everyone seems to have nice things to say about you. I mean, your colleagues in CT surgery don't seem to get along too often, and they usually come complaining to me. But I've noticed that no matter who I talk to—no matter which faction they're from—they seem to think you're all right."

"Mostly," I responded after taking a moment to reflect on a subject that had not previously occurred to me, "I think it's because I just keep myself very busy and try to avoid gossip or taking sides. Maybe it's also because I look for qualities that I really respect in each of my colleagues." That had been my strategy at the university, and also at the San Francisco VA.

Without many problems to discuss, my conversation with Nancy that morning drifted to a variety of topics, and eventually settled on her frustrations in dealing with the operating room politics and interdepartmental struggles at UCSF. Suddenly, she turned to me with what she must have thought was a relatively innocuous question.

"How are things in the OR over at the VA?"

It may have seemed like a simple question, but it hit me like a thunderbolt. In fact, it triggered an epiphany that would alter the course of the remainder of my experience at the VA.

Never having let go of the VA myself, I was suddenly struck by the fact that someone like Nancy, who almost certainly had spent time at a VA during her training, might not have even set foot in a VA facility for decades. Although I had never envied Nancy the political headaches she lamented, all that now paled in comparison to what I realized we dealt with daily at the VA.

Nancy's question forced me to confront the fact that thousands of excellent people—many extremely competent, some recognized world experts in their fields—worked every day at VA hospitals without consciously noting that they were participating in a system that complacently provided mediocre care to our nation's veterans. Though I'm certain none of them had delusions about the place or its collective view of its patients, mediocre care was such an accepted, ingrained component of the VA reality that it simply did not register in their conscious minds. I'm equally certain that most would have said that their contribution to veteran care remained at the highest possible level, without considering the larger picture of the VA patients' experiences as a whole.

That certainly had been true of me. Even after I became a VA staff surgeon, I avoided facing with a clear, open mind the full toxic VA reality. Sure, deep down I knew it was a mediocre institution that provided second-rate care. But I came to work there, did my job as well as I could, fit in to the degree I felt comfortable, and ignored the negative realities.

Although my thoughts had dwelled hundreds of times on both institutions, Nancy's question—likely asked out of innocent curiosity—dropped a bomb in my brain. I had never until that moment let myself so clearly contrast UCSF and the San Francisco VA side by side. I tried not to let Nancy notice how startled I felt, and I calmly told her that things simply "felt different over there" and that it was even harder to get things done than at UC. But I was stunned.

Suddenly, I could no longer ignore the stark differences in standards and expectations that separated the VA from institutions that truly strove to achieve the excellence in patient care that the VA's public relations people trumpeted. Suddenly, I realized how VA assumptions and attitudes blinded the professional staff to the double standard they adopted every time they walked through a door into a VA facility. Suddenly, I realized that there was no justification for yielding to the attitude "C'mon, this is the VA."

* * *

Of course, doctors set the tone and the standards for the medicine practiced in any healthcare system. But in a hospital, much of what the doctors intend can only be delivered to the patients through the competent dedication of a talented nursing staff. As I sat in Nancy Ascher's wood-paneled office at UCSF that morning in 2006, I began to realize exactly how and why the operating rooms at UCSF and the VA differed so dramatically from each other.

The nursing staff in any hospital is not only critical for organizing the OR and making sure that all the systems and processes work, but the nurses also set the mood. In general, the OR nurses at UCSF loved what they did. They were fully aware that although they did not themselves perform the operations, their understanding of the patients and the procedures could have a lasting impact on outcomes. Their professionalism demanded respect, and they were in turn very respectful of the doctors at each level of training.

The OR nurses at UCSF would often talk about gaming the OR schedule, trying to wrangle an assignment to a particular case. They would sometimes joke about their motives (e.g., avoiding the pus that would need to be drained from a peri-rectal abscess), but their real reasons were often career development interests and intellectual drive. Since many nurses had pursued particular specialties (orthopedic surgery, cardiac surgery, urology, and so on) they would often seek out interesting or challenging cases that would allow them to raise their level of performance in their chosen specialty.

Of course there were limits. UCSF nurses belonged to a strong union, and union contracts specified shifts of a set duration—sometimes eight hours, sometimes twelve. Break times had to be respected. When the time came for their meals, nurses were always excused from the operation and replaced by stand-ins. These personnel considerations sometimes caused difficulties, but the UCSF operating rooms never closed. Cases would be scheduled late into the day, or even into the night, and there were always emergency "add-ons" waiting to be assigned to rooms once the last scheduled surgery was done. Nursing shifts were scheduled in anticipation of these inevitable emergencies, and if emergencies exceeded capacity, additional nursing and anesthesia staff were on call to cover the unanticipated need.

Nurses at the VA also frequently tried to influence the operating room schedule. Their overriding concern, however, was almost always to prevent cases from running beyond three o'clock in the afternoon. At three o'clock, all but two of the eight operating rooms at the San Francisco VA were required to be emptied of all personnel and, therefore, no operations were scheduled that might creep beyond that deadline. The remaining two operating rooms were allowed to function until five o'clock, when they, too, were shut down. Shutting down by three o'clock meant that operations had to be wrapped up well before then but, more importantly, surgeries were never scheduled to start beyond an even earlier hour, which meant that it was almost impossible to schedule more than one big operation per day. Since it was common for an hour or more to pass before an operating room was cleaned between cases, and since it was common for the anesthesia team to take an hour to prepare a patient for surgery, no further cases could be contemplated if the previous case was likely to end after one p.m. The needs of patients could rarely compete with these administrative considerations. If wait lists grew longer for critically necessary operations, so be it.

Meanwhile, OR staff were paid for their shift whether they assisted operations or not. Cases were usually slow to start in the morning, and final details were usually wrapped up early. If any doctor sought to influence this program of underutilization, there was heavy resistance. The nursing staff in charge of scheduling made sure that most cases fell within acceptable time boundaries. But if a case that had not yet begun threatened to go "late," the operating room charge nurse, who had responsibility for staffing each case with two nurses, could easily announce, "No, we don't have any nurses available for your case."

And so the key for VA nurses was to get assigned to a first case that would last long enough to prevent a second case from starting. Or to stretch out that first case in the operating room long enough to achieve the same goal.

This limitation on operating room time was a great frustration for my general thoracic surgery service. Not only could our difficult cases take several hours, but thoracic surgery almost always required an unusually long anesthesia preparation. In the hands of skilled anesthesia specialists, this preparation could often be accomplished within thirty or forty minutes. At the VA, it often took two hours or more. Even if a patient made it into the operating room at the first daily OR start time of 7:30 a.m., it was virtually impossible to get a second case started.

My only hope to move more patients off the waiting list and onto the operating table was to find short cases that I knew I could get done in an hour or less, match them up with cases that would more typically take longer, and then arrange for the short cases to go to the OR earlier than the harder ones. But this scheme depended on my getting the shorter case done quickly, so there could be no excuse to shut down my operating room before I started the second case. Yet more often than not, the OR schedulers or the OR nursing staff would switch the order of my cases. My counterattack: more than once, I went to my patient's room at six a.m. and wheeled the patient myself to the pre-op holding area to make sure his surgery time wasn't switched at the last minute.

> "Operating room nurses [at the VA in New York City] refused to allow operations to start after 1 PM for fear of having to stay past 4 PM, when their shifts ended." Facility administrators have also been complicit in the practice, even ensuring surgeons did not take some appointments in the afternoon. "Hospital administrators limited operating time, making sure that work stopped by 3 PM. Consequently, the physician in charge kept a list of patients who needed surgery and rationed the available slots to those with the most urgent problems," wrote one physician of the VA's practices. The result was surgical facilities being rendered nonoperational and patients going without needed care.
>
> –Coburn Report [14]

---

[14] p. 27.

To be fair, there was a progressive effort over the years to get VA operations to start on time—which largely meant getting a patient into the operating room by 7:30 a.m.—likely because that benchmark was something that began to be recorded and reported. Eventually, a stream of angry emails would follow if our residents ever failed to have all the operative consent forms and other paperwork ready for a patient at that appointed time. And yet, any other effort made to get more done in the operating room once the cases "started on time" was resisted tooth and nail. Ostensibly, the explanation for needing to close all but two of the VA ORs by three p.m. (and the remainder by five) was related to budgetary constraints. And yet these constraints never seemed to stop the VA from spending money on things like a virtually useless, million-dollar surgical robot.

> [Claims that such limitations on the provision of care are driven by budgetary concerns were called into question by the fact that] the VA ends nearly every year with tens of billions in unspent funds. This includes at least a half-a-billion dollars specifically intended to provide health care.
>
> –Coburn Report [15]

* * *

Getting patients into the operating room was one hurdle. Getting their cases done well was the next. The eagerness of the UCSF nurses to participate in cutting edge, world-class surgery also meant that they were very interested in what happened on and around the operating table. They watched closely and learned. They anticipated needs. They made sure instruments and equipment were at the ready before they were needed—instruments and equipment that could save time and effort. That time and effort could sometimes save a life.

---

[15] p. 5.

At the VA, on the other hand, I felt lucky whenever I was assigned a nurse who was interested enough in thoracic surgery to come into the OR eager and well prepared. From most of the others I was not greeted by preparation and anticipation, but by blank stares. Though everybody showed up for work at the VA, as was their responsibility, that was about as far as their dedication to excellence often reached.

And then there was the problem of anesthesia. Thoracic anesthesia is itself a complex subspecialty, requiring skills of the anesthesiology team that often takes years to cultivate and to master. In contrast to the dedicated, highly skilled, and specialized thoracic anesthesiologists who helped manage our cases at UCSF, at the VA I was also almost always assigned anesthesiologists who had little or no familiarity with managing the unique challenges of operations within the chest. Once, I had to stop a case at the VA, remove my sterile gloves, and call over to an anesthesia colleague at UCSF so he could coach my VA anesthesiologist through the rest of the case.

Sitting in Nancy Ascher's office that morning in 2006, more than fifteen years after I started working at VA hospitals, I began to think hard for the first time why it was so much more difficult to bring the same level of healthcare to the vets that was expected almost everywhere else in the United States. I realized more clearly than ever that getting patients who needed lifesaving surgery into and out of the operating room was just a greater challenge at the VA than at any of the academic and private hospitals where I had worked during the course of my medical training and early career. But I also realized that surgical care doesn't stop at the operating room door. And for patients like the veterans who bring many other types of healthcare challenges with them into the operating room, the difficult road to complete recovery doesn't end with their discharge from the hospital.

It was true that most patients at UCSF had stronger home situations to which they could return from their stay in the hospital, and that fewer of them needed extra support to make sure that the remainder of their recoveries went well. But when patients did need more (extra care at home or perhaps additional time at an appropriate skilled nursing facility), the UCSF social workers were there to make sure patients continued to receive the very best.

The VA had social workers, too. Many of them seemed to work pretty hard, because almost every vet needed something more to make his or her discharge acceptable. But with the restrictions on VA-approved facilities and services, they had very little to work with. And so, once again, something was almost always considered better than nothing. Even though that something often wasn't very good. Even the best-intentioned social workers were often satisfied to find a place that would simply take in our post-op vets who could not go straight home. Since many vets did not even have a real home, that was a lot of patients. Thoracic patients, as I learned all too well, were among the sickest of the sick, and they often needed even more help than most to get back on their feet. But more important to me, these were *my* patients. And so I found myself struggling over the appropriateness of a discharge plan almost as often as I found myself struggling to get the patients into the hospital in the first place.

More than once, a VA social worker who genuinely cared would thank me quietly in the hallway for being obstinate, and for not agreeing to the plan she had felt forced to advocate.

"Dr. Mann!" a familiar voice called out to me early one chilly San Francisco evening as I walked through the wind from the main hospital building to the parking lot at the VA. It was a familiar voice, yet one I could not immediately place. I turned around to identify the source and was surprised to see our service's very dedicated and almost always cheerful social worker, who was also leaving the hospital fairly late.

"Dr. Mann," she repeated, coming close enough now that she could speak to me in a slightly subdued tone, "I've noticed you don't really belong here at the VA."

I was somewhat startled, but her warm smile made it clear that this was not the beginning of a reprimand.

"Most people manage to fit in here really well, but some people just don't. I've noticed you seem to care too much about what happens to your patients. I really appreciate it every time that you stand up and say 'No!' to one of my discharge plans that really isn't right. You don't seem to mind causing trouble over your patients' welfare. That's not too common around here, and I know it's not very easy."

"You care an awful lot more than average yourself," I said to the woman who had stayed on at the VA despite years of complaints to me, at least in private, about how frustrated she often felt by the constraints under which she was forced to work.

"It's the vets," I pointed out after a slight pause. "You and I are still here because of the vets. We don't want to leave them here by themselves, with no one left to fight for them."

"You're right, Dr. Mann. You're exactly right."

With that, we parted ways for the evening, just a little more comforted by having confirmed our sense of not being entirely alone.

CHAPTER EIGHT

Daniel Harrison

Without intention, and without even realizing what she had done, Nancy Ascher triggered an epiphany in my mind one spring morning in 2006. She prompted me to think clearly, perhaps for the very first time, about the full depth and breadth of the differences between the OR we both knew at UCSF and its counterpart at the San Francisco VA. In doing so, she spurred me to realize more about the entire VA institution.

I had kept my answer to Nancy Ascher's question about the VA ORs relatively simple that morning, but after I left her office, the question festered in my mind. Eventually, it became clearer and clearer to me how the VA did it. How it resisted change, how it resisted improvement. The expectations were so low that anything seemed like an accomplishment. It started with expectations of the patients. They were viewed as impossibly unhealthy, and essentially unable to take better care of themselves. There was no ambition to elevate the general level of veteran health; the challenge at the VA was to patch together these "sicker" patients despite their inevitably bad shape.

But since, to everyone, we were all "at the VA," the low expectations didn't stop with the patients. "This was not the Cleveland Clinic." And it never would be. So "okay" was good enough. Better than nothing was, well, better than nothing.

Without having gone into great detail, I had tried to explain to Nancy that all the foibles and annoyances of UCSF seemed to me a small price to pay for avoiding the indifference of VA OR nursing and the indifferent atmosphere of the entire place. But as my mind raced around the surprisingly startling realizations that her simple question had triggered, it also became clearer and clearer that the most important deficits I faced in my crusade to do more for San Francisco veterans manifested during that part of their care between the operating room suite and discharge.

Many of the most important aspects of successful surgery involve what happens in the days after the patient leaves the OR. At UCSF, the professionalism of the OR nurses was matched by the dedication to excellence we found consistently in the ICU and on the "regular" wards.

The limited number of effective resources at the San Francisco VA had somehow been focused on the immediate postoperative period, and an acceptably competent surgical ICU staff had actually been assembled and trained. The ICU nurses at the San Francisco VA were usually able to help get our patients past the often difficult immediate postoperative period. But once the patients were transferred out of the ICU, good luck. Surgeons from every specialty knew to drag their feet whenever the question came up about transferring post-op patients out of the ICU. After that, it sometimes seemed that patients were on their own. We were often able to keep patients in the ICU until they had recovered enough to be ready to go home.

So although I had spoken to Nancy Ascher about why she should complain a little less about the OR environment at UCSF, it became clear to me that the most stark contrast between the two institutions was really on the regular wards. And although Nancy and I wrapped up our meeting talking about other things, I could not get the face of one veteran in particular, Danny Harrison, out of my mind.

Daniel Harrison was a tough, 250-pound, African-American ex-marine in his early sixties who had a weak heart and needed multiple bypasses. During the many weeks he eventually spent at the San Francisco VA, we heard numerous stories from his family describing the way he had remained their pillar of strength over the years despite his failing health. Mr. Harrison had always prided himself on his physical strength and endurance, and yet it was clear from these stories that it had been compassion and thoughtful insight, rather than intimidation, that characterized the leadership he had provided for his grateful family.

Mr. Harrison was one of those cardiac surgery patients who'd had a "stormy" postoperative course. With a badly weakened heart going into his bypass operation, and a long, difficult case, Mr. Harrison had gone into multi-organ failure in the early postoperative period. For many critically ill patients, that would have been a sign that recovery was impossible. In fact, several ICU staff people began to argue that we should encourage the family to "let him go." But there was something about this ex-marine that spoke to me and told me that he had a least one more battle left in him. And so we nursed his heart off of all the machines and medicine "drips" until it was finally clear that Mr. Harrison would be able to sustain life on his own.

What was not yet clear at that point, however, was whether Mr. Harrison's brain function would recover as well as his heart. In order to allow the patient to rest completely and heal his heart, he had been pharmacologically paralyzed and sedated throughout his early postoperative course. And after all those days of accumulating paralytic agents and sedative drugs, and with kidneys and a liver that were not functioning too well with the stress of this sickness and an inconsistent blood supply, it was not too surprising that even after the drugs were turned off, Mr. Harrison was not too quick to wake up.

But he did finally start to come out of his coma after about another week. We had known early on that even if he survived, it would take many weeks to wean him off the ventilator that had been breathing for him by pushing air into and out of his lungs. And we also knew that the safest and most comfortable way to keep Mr. Harrison on a ventilator for such a prolonged period of time was to create a hole in his neck, called a "tracheostomy," through which the tube connected to the ventilator could be inserted down into his windpipe.

So when Mr. Harrison finally began to wake up, he woke up with a tube coming out of a hole in his neck. That meant that even if he wanted to speak to the multitude of different nurses, doctors, and therapists whom he couldn't possibly have recognized, he wouldn't have been able to make any noise; the tube keeping him alive also funneled each breath away from his voice box and prevented him from uttering a sound.

But I had noticed that even if Mr. Harrison couldn't speak, he was feeling everything that was going on, to him and around him. During the many weeks of Mr. Harrison's struggle, I would find him at times staring out the window of his ICU room. To others, he might have seemed to be in a drug-induced stupor, but I noticed intermittent tears that would well up in the corner of the former marine's eye. I could sense the sheer frustration of this strong man who had become so weak, and who was finding it just too hard to hang on to life.

And so I broke an unspoken rule and allowed myself to become emotionally involved in this patient's care. Not that doctors are supposed to be uncaring, but without a certain ability to detach, it is unlikely that any human being could maintain his or her sanity through hundreds of life and death scenarios, some of which are inevitably, statistically doomed not to end well. But I allowed myself to connect with Mr. Harrison, and I found myself spending hours at his ICU bedside, cheering on his baby steps in weaning from the ventilator, shoring up his courage in the face of the relentless pain, and joining in his determination during the constant uphill struggle just to regain the strength to sit up straight and dangle his legs over the edge of the bed.

Despite the moral support, it was a rocky course for Mr. Harrison. He required placement of a pacemaker to keep his heart from beating too slowly. The stress also took an irreversible toll on his kidneys, and among the many tubes that went in and out of his body during this prolonged ordeal were catheters that would allow him to be connected to an artificial kidney machine to clean his blood.

But finally, against all odds, and against the expectations of just about every member of the ICU staff, Mr. Harrison was weaned from the ventilator. With a lot of help from the physical therapists, and with an unbridled determination to recover, he was even able to support his own weight and, leaning heavily on a walker, to take a few small steps. He still needed to be hooked back up to the ventilator for stretches at night, and he often needed a little help suctioning thick mucus that would plug up the tracheostomy tube in his neck. That degree of support, however, could be provided on the San Francisco VA step-down unit, and so Mr. Harrison was transferred out of the ICU.

Although the nurses on Ward 3B complained quite a bit initially about the level of work involved in his care, Mr. Harrison's sparkling eyes and his irresistible smile won them over. In fact, things went pretty smoothly during his predictably long wait for a bed at one of the few facilities to which veterans could be sent for long-term rehabilitation from ventilatory support while also on dialysis. And so I was surprised one day to hear that a problem involving Mr. Harrison had come to interrupt the normal flow of morning rounds.

"I think we ought to start rounds with Mr. Harrison," was the greeting I received that morning from the intern on the CT Surgery Service

"Mr. Harrison?" I asked in genuine surprise. "Mr. Harrison's on 3B. We always start rounds here in the ICU."

Rounds normally started at the location within the hospital that housed the patients with the highest acuity. On the Cardiothoracic Service that almost always meant the intensive care unit. It was a form of triage, and it made perfect sense. So it was a strange suggestion for rounds to begin instead at Mr. Harrison's bedside on Ward 3B.

"I know," the more seasoned, second-year resident on the service jumped in. "But I also think you had better hear about this first."

I became both anxious and a little angry.

"If something's wrong with Mr. Harrison," I said sternly as my friendly morning smile quickly dissipated, "I should have been called."

"Things just sort of unfolded right before pre-rounds," the second-year resident continued, "and by then it seemed we should just wait to discuss it in person."

I did not at all like the sound of what I was hearing, but I decided to let the junior residents have their way. If anything truly bad had happened to Mr. Harrison just before rounds, I reassured myself, there would likely still have been a "code blue" resuscitation going on instead of this relatively calm discussion. If something bad had happened earlier in the night, the patient would have been transferred back to the ICU, so needing to go to Ward 3B was actually a good sign. I instructed the intern to tell me what was going on as we walked down the third floor hallway away from the ICU.

"Well," the young doctor began, "the last nursing note we found on Mr. Harrison was from about one a.m. Apparently his TV was still on, and so his nurse went into the room and asked him if he wanted her to turn it off. She indicated in her note that he ignored her questions, so she just let him keep watching the TV."

The team turned the corner of the large hospital corridor as the intern continued on with his somewhat hesitant narrative.

"Apparently, a little after two a.m., the nursing assistant went into his room. She told the nurse that he had fallen asleep, so she turned off the TV."

I tried to hide my exasperation, instead encouraging the surgical trainee to get to the point.

"At about five thirty or five forty-five, the nursing assistant went back into his room one more time, this time to take his vitals, which she apparently hadn't taken during the entire shift . . ."

The intern paused again. We were now standing at the entrance to Ward 3B. Through the reinforced glass of the large doors to the ward's central corridor, I could see the hospital's director of nursing services huddled over the counter of the main nursing station, in an animated discussion with the charge nurse on duty.

"Yes?" I found it necessary to prod the young first-year resident one last time. "And what were his vitals?"

"Mr. Harrison was dead."

I had heard the young man clearly, but his unexpected words reverberated in my head without really registering. In confusion, I instinctively turned to the older resident to explain to me what the intern had said.

"When we looked back at the strips from his EKG monitor," the second-year resident jumped in, "we realized he must have died just before midnight."

I felt an awful, familiar gnawing in my gut. Despite my many years of training, I had still not gotten used to losing a patient. But of all the nonsense I had heard, or heard about, in those many years of rotating through numerous hospitals, this was perhaps the most ridiculous tragedy I had ever been asked to swallow.

"What?!" I was a little too stunned to be angry. "How is that even possible? I thought he was on the monitor?"

"That's what we all thought at first." The intern was now eager to run through the detective work that had filled his time just before rounds. "So we looked back at the strips. Even though his EKG was flatline, his pacemaker kept firing after he died, and the monitor interpreted that as a QRS and so the alarms never went off.

"I asked them to pull up the records of the entire shift's EKG tracings," he continued, emboldened at having finally captured all of my concentrated attention, "and Mr. Harrison had had his normal EKG at 11 p.m. By 11:15 his heart rate dropped below 50, and that's when his pacer kicked in and started firing for the rest of the night. Finally, about 11:50, he stopped responding altogether to the pacer and soon he deteriorated into V-tach, then V-fib. By midnight everything except the pacer spike was flat."

"And you're saying the monitor never alarmed because it interpreted the pacing spike as the patient's own heartbeat?" I had heard and understood the explanation, but I repeated it simply because I had never before encountered a scenario in which an electronic device was the only means of knowing whether the signal on an EKG monitor reflected the discharge of electricity from a pacemaker or the beat of a human heart.

"But why weren't the nurses looking at the monitors themselves? How could they not have seen what was going on?"

When the news first hit, I had succumbed for an instant to the instinctual hope that somehow there had been a terrible mistake, that somehow I might find dear Mr. Harrison still alive, still smiling somewhere on Ward 3B. But the stark reality of what I was being told left no room for denial. Faced with the facts, as absurd as they might be, both my junior residents and I already knew the answer to these two obvious questions.

It would not take long even for a recent medical school graduate to perceive the difference between the qualified, professional nurses who populated the wards at the university hospital and the general level of nurses who ended up settling for employment at the VA.

So the team simply stood at the entrance to Ward 3B and looked at each other, as the team had no inclination to put into words the obvious answers to my two near-rhetorical questions. First, it was very plausible that the nurses had not been looking at the monitors. I could imagine them asking themselves: Why spend hours staring at a bunch of screens with EKG tracings that almost never change? These were run-of-the-mill VA nurses, not the ones who had somehow been recruited to our uncharacteristically competent ICU. And for them, there were so many other, more interesting things to do with their time. There was gossip, and there were magazines. There was heating up little delicious home-made delicacies in the microwave oven in the lounge and sharing them with friends. There was running through the upcoming shift schedules, and analyzing who were getting the vacations they requested and who were signing up for extra shifts. These were the things I would routinely find the VA nurses doing at night when I went rounding on the sickest patients. So there would have been many more interesting things for these nurses to do besides staring at telemetry screens with EKG traces that almost never changed.

And besides—and this was really the crucial point—if anything ever went wrong, they assumed, the monitors would alarm and inform them of the problem.

So it really was no mystery why the EKG traces of the patients on this monitored step-down unit at the San Francisco VA had not actually been monitored by the nurses as they would have been monitored in a similar ward at UCSF.

But my other rhetorical question was just as telling. Because even if the nurse assigned to the monitors had been looking at them, it was still quite possible that she might not have known what was going on. It was quite possible that she wouldn't have recognized the abnormal slowing down of the patient's heart. In retrospect, the slowing of Mr. Harrison's heart had almost certainly been the first sign of a mucus plug that had clogged up his tracheostomy tube, preventing him from getting the oxygen his heart needed despite being hooked up to a machine that was providing a minimal degree of support for his natural breaths. A mucus plug that could so easily have been suctioned right out of that tracheostomy without causing Mr. Harrison any harm. If only the suction catheter had been left within Mr. Harrison's reach, as it should have been.

Or if only a competent nurse had noticed something amiss with his EKG tracing at any time during the forty-five minutes it took him to die, and had bothered to walk the fifteen feet into his room to see what was wrong.

Even without the ability to suction himself, though, Mr. Harrison would have had time early on to call to the nurses for help. Whether Mr. Harrison had tried to ring the call button for help as his distress began to mount, or whether in his still infirm state he couldn't find or reach the call button that the nurses should have made sure was easily within his reach, I would never know. Since the distress must have begun for Mr. Harrison just at around the time of the eleven o'clock change of shift, when nurses were preoccupied with giving each other reports on the patients and hated being interrupted, I suspected that if the call button had been rung, it might very well have been ignored.

So the answers to my first two questions were better left unspoken, but after a little more incredulous thought, I still had a few more things to ask.

"And what about the visits to his room? You're telling me that a registered nurse went into my dead patient's room, asked him if he wanted her to turn off the TV, and when my dead patient 'ignored' her question, she was so offended that she decided to let him keep watching the TV?"

Yes, everyone on the team agreed in silence, this really was a bit hard to believe.

"And then you're telling me that a trained nursing assistant went back an hour later, saw my dead patient slumped over in his bed, and turned off his TV so that it wouldn't wake him up?"

After a few more uncomfortably silent moments, it was pretty obvious to everyone on cardiothoracic surgery rounds that there was nothing more to be said about Mr. Harrison's demise. There would be forms to fill out and more questions that did need to be answered later, but right now it was also obvious that the director of nursing was running "damage control" from the ward.

Bad things happen everywhere. Plenty of mistakes were made over at UCSF Medical Center; they had been made during my time at Harvard's Brigham and Women's Hospital, and at Stanford Hospital, too. But Mr. Harrison's death at the VA was not the same. It was not just a matter of human error in the pursuit of excellence.

Everyone at the VA knew that there was an enormous drop in nursing acumen on the regular wards. Everyone knew that there was a reason why patients were kept an inordinate amount of time in the ICU. This was the case in San Francisco, and it had been the case in Palo Alto and in Boston, where I had spent time in similarly "high-quality" VAs. The real problem was this: this situation, this below-par performance, was all considered acceptable, and was accepted. This was the VA. The expectation was for care that could never reach the level of centers like UCSF. It was part of a nationwide culture that persisted unscathed past the much-touted VA transformation of the 1990s.

Mr. Harrison could have survived at a place like UCSF, but his survival was simply unlikely at the VA. I mulled things over one more time, then turned my team around and started leading them back down the hall toward the ICU.

"Let's go round," I said to the people I was responsible for training. "And let's hope that some of our other patients are still alive."

> In Ohio, Air Force veteran Charles Pennington bled to death following a liver biopsy, because hospital staff did not check in on him after his procedure.
>
> —Coburn Report [16]

---

[16] p. 19.

CHAPTER NINE

"The Harder You Push, the Slower I'll Go"

It was not just benign neglect. Somehow, that might have been more tolerable. Instead, the VA actively resisted change—people at the VA actively resisted change. Not everyone. Most of the part-time physicians would have been happy to see things improve, to find it easier to get things done for their VA patients. But many members of the full-time staff had paid a price, had discarded professional goals, had sacrificed self-esteem, had accepted lower salary scales, had abandoned career ambitions of excellence and distinction. And so, in exchange for these sacrifices, a bargain needed to be kept by the VA devil. One of those benefits was the promise of a slow, lazy pace of work. For these people, a demand for hard work was inconceivable. And not to be tolerated.

Even after I had left my 2006 career-development meeting with Nancy Ascher, I was haunted by the feeling that I had not yet put my finger squarely on the biggest difference between the operating rooms at UCSF and the OR at the San Francisco VA. I imagined myself in both places, and it was as if I were imagining two different selves. One was relaxed and yet excited, filled with eager anticipation. The other was apprehensive, on guard, oppressed.

Then it hit me.

The OR at UCSF was like every other operating room of my surgical education and training. It was a place where the pagers were turned off (or at least passed off to someone else), and where the usual din of beckoning problems and annoyances were replaced by a brief interval of Zen-like calm focus on a single undertaking. Where skills could be honed and practiced in a supportive environment, among respected friends and allies. And where there was always a sense that you were making a big difference in someone's life. During my residency at Harvard, one of my attendings had once described surgery as the only profession that allowed grown-ups to come to work, put on their pajamas, and play.

The atmosphere in VA operating rooms, in stark contrast, reflected the bitterness and general malcontent that characterized the rest of the hospital. Many of the nurses were no more excited to be there than their counterparts on the wards, and the anesthesiologists certainly did not feel any deep sense of professional satisfaction at having "made it to the VA." But it wasn't just discontent and bitterness. As I contrasted the atmospheres of the two ORs, I realized that poison hung in the sanitized air of the VA operating rooms. It was not just discontent; it was malice.

I had heard of the backstabbing long before I had experienced any of it. Michael Baker's warning of OR lounge gossip one morning had caught me off guard, but it did not throw me for a loop. Gossip, and even warnings, that I had heard from other surgeons lent credibility to Michael's admonition. The OR nursing and technologist staff had a weapon with which they could threaten any one of either the part-time or even the "eight-eighths" VA surgeons: any of us could get "written up," any time, for almost any reason. There were formal incident reports and less formal complaints. But none of these write-ups could be ignored. Some might lead to sanctions, others to more serious disciplinary actions. The great irony of this weapon was that the surgeons had much less of an opportunity to complain. The nurses and other staff members were protected by stringent union rules and VA employment policies.

Not so for the doctors. Criticism from below could have a searing, penetrating impact, and part-time physicians were categorized as "temporary" by VA legislation, which meant they had no legal job protection whatsoever. Colleagues of mine had often mentioned being hauled in and questioned over accusations of inappropriate and unprofessional intimidation or abuse of OR staff members. Foul language, "public disparagement"—these would comprise serious transgressions. Harassment of medical students was a common incrimination, raised only a minority of times by the students themselves. But throwing instruments in the operating room was one of the absolute favorite charges. To be sure, my colleagues were not all angels, but for the most part their professionalism was, in my experience, beyond reproach. The accusation of "unprofessional behavior," however, was particularly menacing. Not only could it be grounds for dismissal from the VA component of one's employment, it could actually become the grounds for suspension or revocation of one's license to practice medicine.

An awareness of this very uncharacteristic and uncomfortable aspect of the OR atmosphere at the VA seeped slowly into one's consciousness. But how had it evolved? At the surface, there seemed to be a simple enjoyment of watching others squirm that may have stemmed simply from the general malcontent of people who worked for the VA. It was a generally oppressive and fearful environment, and apprehensive people tend to gain some comfort from any opportunity to exert some control over their unpredictable environment. Even if that control amounted to little more than gratuitous "professional violence." And, of course, it could be an outlet for their own frustration and pent-up aggression.

But over time I realized that there was a more Machiavellian possibility, as well.

The threat of recrimination kept doctors in their place. It provided a weapon against the occasional attempt to bring more or harder work into the OR. Perhaps most importantly, it provided a strong disincentive against stirring up trouble over substandard performances. Why rock the boat—why complain about any one incompetent individual—if it was almost impossible to buck the enormous trend of VA mediocrity? And especially if the most likely result was that you alone would end up in the water without a life jacket.

A year or two had gone by since my joining the VA staff before I experienced my first write-up. The case in question had seemed benign enough. We were in the midst of one of the most sensitive and difficult components of a coronary bypass operation, and I asked my scrub nurse for a particular type of clamp, an instrument for holding suture needles and driving them through the patient's tissues. I was handed the wrong one, and I quickly passed it back and explained what I needed in its place. A few moments later, I asked again for the same instrument and was again passed the wrong version of the needle-holding clamp. When this happened a fourth time, I realized the only way I could avoid this time-consuming and disruptive hiccup was to remove the incorrect instrument from the sterile operating field altogether. And so I turned from the table, lowered my hand, and dropped the incorrect needle-driver on the unsterile floor.

"You've been accused of throwing an instrument" was the way Mark Ratcliffe summed up the incident report that followed as I sat in his office several days later.

"What are you talking about?" My surprise, as well as my confusion, was genuine.

"The circulator and the scrub nurse both verified that, in a fit of anger, you threw a needle-driver across the room during Wednesday's bypass."

I remembered that moment of the operation clearly. It had been an unconventional move on my part, but it had been done quietly, without ceremony, without any outburst, and without any ill intent. Importantly, it had had its exact intended positive effect on the flow of the operation— from that moment on, I was handed the correct instruments. I began to explain to Mark why I had simply dropped the needle-driver on the OR floor. Mark waved his hand, indicating that the words were both a waste of my breath and a waste of his time.

"The circulator reported that the instrument travelled so far across the room and landed with such a force that when it hit the ground, the patient's blood splashed up and hit him in the eye."

If there had been an ounce of truth to this tale, this last bit of over-reaching should have undermined any of its credibility.

"The thing never touched the patient's body. It was the wrong instrument that I had been handed several times. It couldn't have had any blood on it—certainly not enough to 'splash' anyone in the eye."

"Michael Baker was in the room, and he has confirmed the whole thing. There's no point to arguing; it just indicates a lack of insight. I'll need a written explanation and an apology, and I'll try to get you off with just a warning. Maybe some anger management training."

That uncontrolled anger had been implicated as my motive was a very significant, aggravating element in the accusation. If I had raised my voice as part of a thoughtful, calculated attempt to induce better discipline and improve performance in the operating theater, my methods could have been questioned, but there would be substance for debate. The loss of control to unfettered emotion, on the other hand, would have been inherently unprofessional and an inexcusable, unjustifiable offense.

The most elegant and insidiously impregnable component of the indictment, however, was Ratcliffe's offhanded reference to a "lack of insight." The accusation of "lacking insight" aggravated any offense at the VA and ratcheted up the degree of discipline required in the response. The words not only obliterated any opportunity for clarification or self-vindication, they rendered any attempt at such worse than useless. It actually became additional fodder for profound self-incrimination.

The scrub nurse on the case was a fairly regular participant in the "heart room," but was not a member of our "A-team." The circulator, on the other hand, was one of the core cardiac nurses, and therefore someone with whom I had worked closely for some time. We had never previously had any suggestion of conflict, nor had I sensed any animosity in our frequent, friendly exchanges. It was therefore disheartening that this individual had chosen to participate in an attack on my character and my standing in the VA OR. But still, he was someone I did not know all that well.

My real disillusionment came with the mention of Michael Baker's name. Ever since his assignment as nurse manager of the general thoracic operating room upon my appointment to the San Francisco VA staff in 2003, we had worked closely to build a respectable program. We had faced frequent adversities, and we had grown to trust each other to do the right thing. We had relied on each other many times, and although we had never socialized in any way, I had considered the man my friend.

Had there been truth to the accusation of my throwing an instrument, I would have hoped that Michael would have come to me before contributing to this type of escalation. But his "confirmation" of such obviously contrived elements as the "uncontrolled anger" and the splashing of fictitious blood (which introduced the further exacerbation of direct bodily harm to the OR staff) indicated that this had not simply been an administrative judgment call on Michael's part. Regardless of whatever mutual respect and professional camaraderie had developed between him and me over the years, Michael had gone ahead when called upon and participated in this VA ritual at my direct expense. I was stunned.

Policy prohibited me from addressing this issue directly with any of my accusers, and so I could only guess at the incentive behind the calumny. At first, it remained a mystery, but as I reflected on the warnings I had gotten from time to time and on similar instances of exaggerated or fictionalized incident reports about which I had been told, a couple of potential motives emerged. Although I had not, in fact, expressed any anger during the case, my frustration with the nurse's performance must have been obvious. Her confusion had come at such a sensitive, potentially life-threatening part of the procedure that it might have seemed possible, if not actually likely, that I would bring this performance issue to someone's attention. The immediate filing of the instrument-throwing incident report neutralized any threat to the nurse's standing because any complaint I made at that point would be viewed as retaliatory (and, not insignificantly, reflective of a lack of insight).

In this one instance, this routine filing of a preemptive incident report had, in fact, effectively neutralized any potential threat to the institution's deeply rooted, though unspoken, acceptance and perpetuation of mediocrity.

> Echoing wider problems across the VA health care system, [Dr. Jeff] Hawker said there is a "climate of fear" at the Salem [Virginia] VA, with many employees looking the other way when they see something wrong for fear of reprisals. After Hawker started reporting unsafe practices, he said one medical technician interrupted him when he brought up a concern. "She said, 'Dr. Hawker, don't tell me anything – the less I know (the better). I just want to be able to retire,'" he recalled.
>
> *–Stars and Stripes* [17]

---

[17] Heath Druzin, "Doctor Says 'Sham Peer Review' Used to Destroy His Career After Pointing Out VA Problems," Stars and Stripes, December 15, 2014, accessed January 25, 2015, http://www.stripes.com/news/veterans/doctor-says-sham-peer-review-used-to-destroy-his-career-after-pointing-out-va-problems-1.319484.

∗ ∗ ∗

This first incident report also came at a time when I had been pushing hard to bring more general thoracic cases into the OR. I was struggling on a weekly basis to get two cases scheduled on thoracic days, and then to actually get the two cases done. I couldn't help but feel that the slap of this concocted but incontrovertible incident report was a reminder of the enormity of the system I was up against, and its resistance to being asked to do more.

The need I felt to get more done, however, was part of a mounting sense of frustration. I had been bringing challenging cases to the OR, and I was part of an increasingly comprehensive, multi-specialty approach to lung cancer at the San Francisco VA. But we simply had not made as much progress as I had hoped toward bringing the same level of lung cancer care to San Francisco vets that patients routinely experienced at UCSF and other top-notch, private centers. One of the greatest frustrations was that our waiting list was still routinely twenty or more patients long, and the resulting backlog for major thoracic surgery was still a good six weeks or longer. A big part of that last problem was the allotment of just three days of OR time per month for general thoracic surgery and the treatment of lung cancer. Three days per month for the single greatest cancer killer in the developed world—in a patient population dominated by elderly current and former smokers.

The VA patient population and the VA administrative system made this already obvious incongruity even worse. The complexity of the patients' baseline health conditions, the weakness of the social and medical support systems, the generally ineffective channels of communication with patients, and the instability of many of our vets' living situations made it fairly common for there to be a last-minute cancellation. If we had had operating room time every day or at least every other day, we might have been able to switch around cases and move something up so that the OR time would not have been wasted so frequently. But with the next case scheduled a week or more away, it was often impossible to juggle patient schedules at the last minute to meet our unexpected needs.

And as a result of these cancellations, we were left, on average, with even *fewer* than three days of OR time per month. But no matter how strong a case I made and no matter how many statistics I brought to bear, my requests for additional OR block time fell on deaf ears.

✱ ✱ ✱

The pervasive resistance to additional work did not seem limited to the OR scheduling committee or the OR schedulers or even the nurses running the OR suite on any given day. There seemed to be resistance at every turn and every level. Nor was the resistance limited to general thoracic cases. If two cases were to get done, things needed to move quickly off the blocks at seven thirty a.m. The first case needed to get in and out of the OR, and the room needed to be cleaned (or "turned over") with enough time left in the day to allow the second patient to be wheeled into the room. A glitch anywhere in that sequence threatened the entire enterprise.

One day, I was hoping to get a couple of important cardiac cases done. At seven forty-five, I meandered into the OR to see how preparations were progressing. The operating room was devoid of human life. As I rushed to the pre-op holding area, where I hoped both to find the patient and to jumpstart the day myself, I literally ran into the anesthesia attending who had been assigned to my room.

"So what's up, John?" I asked in as non-confrontational a voice as I could muster. "Why aren't we in the room?"

"Listen, Mann, I know you've posted a second case, but that's not going to change the way we get things done around here."

"I'm just trying to be helpful." I had already learned that it was best to avoid direct confrontation wherever possible. "I'm just wondering what else needs to get done."

"I need to have an echo machine in the room for this case. I'm not bringing the patient in until I know I have it there. I'm going to check on that now."

This particular reason for delay seemed a bit odd, since the OR had dedicated echo machines that were always kept ready. As my anesthesiologist wandered off, I made my way directly to the storage area where I knew the machine would be waiting. There was no one in the small room, but I found that, in anticipation of its use, everything had been packed up neatly on the mobile device. The machine was about the size of a medium-sized filing cabinet on wheels, so once I had figured out how to unlock the wheels, I began to steer the heavy piece of equipment into the hallway and toward the operating room that had been designated for our case.

I was about halfway down the hall when the attending anesthesiologist began to approach from the opposite direction. He did not look happy. As our paths collided, he put his arms around the echo machine, stopping it dead in its tracks. The fluffy, gossamer, bouffant hair covering on his head did little to dissipate the intimidating anger that was manifested on his face. As he spoke, he made sure to look me straight in the eye.

"Listen, Mann, I know what you're trying to do. Just back off. I'm telling you this, but I'm only going to tell you once: the harder you push, the slower I'll go."

> In New York City, "anesthesiologists routinely cancelled surgeries for personal reasons," said one former VA physician.
>
> –Coburn Report [18]

* * *

Finding a slot in the OR schedule was only the last step in getting a patient off of our pre-op waiting lists. It generally took weeks or months from the moment of referral until the various elements of a patient's work-up had gotten done. These were work-ups that would normally take a week or so at UCSF. But at the VA it took time to get scans, and it took time to get referrals to other services when they were needed for complex patients.

One frequent holdup for many of our patients, strangely, was getting evaluations from the nonsurgical heart doctors, or cardiologists, for patients who needed lung cancer surgery. A history of cigarette smoking, present in roughly 80 percent of American lung cancer patients, was also a major risk factor for heart disease—heart disease that might not yet have been diagnosed, but that could be fatal if discovered during or

---

[18] p. 27.

just after an operation. For that reason, we evaluated the hearts of all of our lung cancer patients prior to subjecting them to stressful and dangerous chest surgeries. And for that, we needed the help of cardiologists.

Cardiology clinic, unfortunately, was so understaffed and so overtaxed at the San Francisco VA, we were told, that we often had to wait many weeks for a clinic appointment while our patients waited for surgery, hoping that the cancer would not spread and progress from curable to incurable during the wait. Since it also took weeks to get other tests done in preparation for surgery, you might ask, why not schedule the cardiology clinic appointment while we were waiting for all the other tests, so that evaluations at least proceeded in parallel? Unfortunately, the cardiologist in charge of these pre-op "clearances" refused to schedule a pre-op patient until we had finished all the other tests and confirmed that the patient was in fact going to have surgery—and was already on the operating room schedule.

After years of struggling with the Catch-22 of pre-op cardiology clearance, the cardiologist in charge finally offered to dedicate two slots in cardiology clinic on my thoracic clinic days so that patients who lived at a great distance and who were likely to need lung cancer surgery could get seen on the same day that they saw me. I leapt at this opportunity, even though the "two slots" were both with nurses, not a real cardiologist—the real cardiologist promised "to see some of these patients, if possible."

* * *

Radiology tests, and in particular a certain test called a "PET scan," were another frequent source of work-up frustration, as the scheduling was haphazard and miscommunication often resulted in missed appointments and additional weeks of delay. The PET scan was a problem because it took years for one to be installed at our medical center—even after it had become a standard of care—and getting anything done outside of a VA facility (for which the VA would need to spend additional money) was even harder than getting things done inside the institution.

But sometimes, getting a particular test done was only half the battle. It might be just as hard to get a qualified doctor to provide an interpretation. That was the case one evening as I repeatedly prodded my team to track down the results of an MRI scan of a certain patient's bones that we suspected might harbor metastatic cancer. It had been a struggle to get the patient on the OR schedule, and although the concern about the bones had been raised some time before, it was just the day before surgery that the MRI had finally gotten done. A positive indication of metastasis would have forced us to delay or cancel the case, since it would likely have made the lung surgery futile. Simply delaying the start of the case was a bad idea, since I had learned the hard way never to allow the VA OR any excuse to push a case off the day's schedule entirely.

The MRI had gotten done; the raw data were sitting somewhere in the VA radiology computer system. But the data needed interpretation from an expert radiologist. Frustrated with my team's acceptance that a "final read" was still not available, I decided to break with protocol and to call the radiology resident myself. At that point in the day—it was already close to eight p.m. at that point—she was the only person listed as "on call" for the VA. That person, however, insisted to me that she was not herself qualified to read an MRI, and that she could not find anyone else to help her interpret the complex test.

"Well, who is your attending on call?" I asked the relatively junior radiology resident. She was on a rotation at the VA that was part of her UCSF residency program. "Why don't we just give that attending a call?"

It would have been a violation of hospital etiquette for us to go over the resident's head and speak directly to her attending before she had had a chance to do so. But I had already deviated from strict protocol by calling the resident myself. Communication was generally maintained at parallel levels of responsibility—residents spoke with residents; attendings spoke with attendings. Although I was very willing to offend this resident if necessary to get an answer for my patient, at that point I was really just enlisting some simple troubleshooting skills to help her get her own job done.

"I've looked through all the lists, and I just can't find anyone."

In a way, I should not have been completely surprised with this answer. The first thing any resident usually does when confronted with a task beyond his or her ability is to look for help. It should not have been surprising that this resident had already searched for an attending. And if she could have found someone easily, we would have had our answer long before I had gotten frustrated enough to give her a call myself.

"I think they maybe forgot to put someone on call."

Given everything I knew about and had experienced at the VA, this should not have been hard to believe either. What *was* extremely hard to believe, however, was that everyone seemed to think this was a perfectly good reason not to get anything done.

"You're kidding" was my kneejerk response. "What would you do if you were faced with an emergency?"

"I'm not sure."

The prolonged pause on her end of the phone betrayed her lack of realization that "I'm not sure" is simply not an acceptable response by a physician to an emergency. But since the pause on her end was not showing any signs of yielding to more constructive comments, I decided to approach the conundrum from a different angle. "Is there a fellow on call who might know which attendings are at least available, even if they're not officially on call?"

"No. Not for the VA. It's just me. I'm the only one on call."

"And you're not able to give me a read on this MRI?"

"No. I'm not prepared to interpret that kind of study."

When most people hit a brick wall at a place like the VA, they simply give up. If one remains determined, however, to do right by a patient, one must either find an existing breach in the wall, or enlist a battering ram.

"All right. Well, who's in charge? Who is the attending who runs your entire service?"

This was now definitive escalation, but leaving a service like radiology completely unstaffed, even for one evening, seemed a good enough excuse.

"I don't know. I guess that would be Dr. Jones. But I definitely wouldn't call him."

"Why not?"

"He really doesn't like to be disturbed."

"Oh, on the contrary," I offered in a friendly, avuncular tone of voice, "I think he would want to know right away if there was a serious problem on his service that was impeding good patient care. I would certainly want to know immediately if there were this type of problem on the Thoracic Service."

"Uh, I really don't think so."

"Well, who else is there? Can you think of another radiologist who can take responsibility for this confusion?"

"No. Just Dr. Jones."

Unlike this poor radiology resident, I did not live in fear of the imposing Dr. Jones. As soon as I said goodbye to the resident, I had the VA operator page Dr. Jones to my cell.

To his credit, Dr. Jones answered the call within several minutes. But the resident couldn't have been more right. He was irate at having been disturbed. He was livid. He wanted to know who the hell I thought I was, and he wanted to know what the hell gave me the right to summon him in this manner.

"I am certainly sorry to bother you after hours," I countered, "but the resident was quite sure that there had been a problem with the scheduling—and that there is no radiology attending listed on call for the VA. I'm taking a patient to the operating room at seven thirty in the morning for a thoracotomy that would be a dangerous mistake if he's got bony metastases. I just need a qualified person to look at the MRI and tell me yes or no."

Dr. Jones had a few more choice words, including the certitude that he would have me held responsible for my insolence in calling him. But, again to his bizarre credit, he agreed to look at the MRI from his computer at home. Eventually, he assured me that the patient's bones were free of cancer.

And to Mark Ratcliffe's credit, when Dr. Jones followed through on his threat, Mark helped to keep the chief of staff, Diana Nicoll, from punishing me for this offense.

* * *

Bureaucratic non sequiturs grew even more contorted as time went by. In 2006, new VA regulations recognized that for many part-time physicians, it was unreasonable or counterproductive to ask them to adhere to a regular weekly tour of duty. The new approach, poetically entitled the "Part-Time Physicians on Adjustable Work Hours" program, required these physicians instead to sign a "Memorandum of Service Level Expectations" delineating how many hours they would work at the VA over the course of a year. They would continue to log their hours each week as worked, but there were no longer strict requirements for certain specific hours to be worked at the VA. In fact, the part-time physicians no longer even needed to log any particular *number* of hours each pay period or each month; at the end of the year, the numbers simply had to add up to what had been promised in his or her own Memorandum of Service Level Expectations. The revised VA Handbook, the VA administrative bible, explained that a representative tour of duty would be noted in ETA (the electronic system into which weekly hours were logged) that reflected the *average* number of hours to be worked per pay period based on the total annual time commitment, but that the actual hours logged could vary freely without the need for any prior approvals.

The whole thing seemed uncharacteristically rational for the VA bureaucracy. Except for one detail: the VA neglected to alter its auditing system to accommodate these very rational changes in procedure. Whomever the time and attendance auditors reported to continued to assign the auditors to the same appointed rounds, and the auditors therefore continued to show up at the same hospitals hunting for errant part-time physicians who were not sitting where they were supposed to be sitting according to a presumed tour of duty.

So, hospital administrators continued to treat the "representative" tours of duty as sacrosanct, even for "Part-Time Physicians on Adjustable Work Hours" who were no longer supposed to adhere to tours of duty. And timekeepers continued to wring their hands and dread the appearance of an auditor at a moment when a part-time physician was not sitting at a desk at which he was no longer obligated to be sitting.

Now that was the VA.

* * *

Over time, I also noticed that checklists became an increasing obsession with VA administrators. What's wrong with checklists? Nothing, if they are relied upon as safety nets to prevent oversights. At the VA, however, people became dependent on them. It was much easier to run through a checklist than to think critically and comprehensively about how to treat a patient, or about the details you may have overlooked or forgotten. Ask any older person who uses GPS why they know less now than in the past about local geography. Being told exactly what to do every time is not conducive to independent analysis or understanding. Ask anyone who has successfully cared for incredibly complex cases in an intensive care unit, and it becomes obvious that no two cases of critical human disease are exactly alike or can possibly be managed "perfectly" by a rigid approach that can be reduced to a number of "checks" on a list, or directives on a computer screen.

However, if the VA had long ago relinquished hope that it could draw into its hospitals those "best minds" in American medicine who could truly perform better without checklists, it had to install additional mechanisms to protect itself from the lower levels of performance by the staff they did attract who could easily miss important details.

Guidelines and standardized pathways are sometimes considered valuable because they eliminate the need to think. And thinking always seemed to make the VA leadership anxious. Perhaps because it seemed scary to be *required* to think, especially under pressure, especially in an emergency.

Perhaps it seemed even scarier to supervise people who were used to thinking for themselves.

* * *

And while the general level of care remained unchanged, enormous amounts of administrative energy were poured into the management of a very few, very specific aspects of our patients' care. For example, a "nurse quality manager" was assigned to make sure that the blood sugar level of every patient who underwent a bypass operation was within a certain acceptable range at six a.m. on the morning after surgery. Derangement of blood sugar levels was okay if it was at five a.m. or at seven, but they had to be spot on at six. If the blood sugars of any fresh post-op patient were off at five o'clock, a resident was expected to be at that patient's bedside manipulating insulin doses and blood sugar levels until the number was exactly right. Then he would need to make sure that no one dared measure the blood sugar again until after 6. If the blood sugar was a little high at 5:55, but then was perfect again at 6:20, there would be hell to pay.

One other detail about our surgical patients suddenly began to get a lot of administrative attention. Patient's nostrils absolutely, positively had to be swabbed upon admission to screen for a certain species of resistant bacterium. There were endless emails about how important it was to make sure blood glucose levels were okay on the last blood glucose measurement before six a.m., and that every nose had been swabbed on admission.

Was getting the blood glucose number to look perfect as close as possible to six a.m. and knowing about the bacteria in the patient's nose on admission really the most important parts of a patient's recovery from heart surgery? More important than whether or not they needed the infusion of powerful drugs, as they often did, to maintain heart function? More important than their ability to maintain good kidney and liver function?

Probably not, but we never got any emails about any of those things.

To be sure, there was some concrete benefit to our patients to have at least one good blood sugar level during their recovery from an enormously complicated operation, and identifying resistant bacteria upon admission to a hospital can't be a bad thing, either. But there was no concerted administrative effort expended at making sure that any of the plethora of other, many much more critical, details of patients' care were falling within an "acceptable" range. Why so much effort just on six a.m. blood glucoses and on nasal swabs for methicillin-resistant *Staphylococcus aureus*?

Who knew? That, too, was the VA way.

* * *

As realizations and frustrations mounted, why did I continue to split my time between UCSF and the VA? Why didn't I take Nancy Ascher up on her implicit, standing offer simply to bring me back to the "mother ship" full time? My professional life had certainly gone well at UCSF, both in the operating room and in my scientific research. Salary support from the VA was therefore no longer an issue, and I had developed an expertise in "beating heart" bypass that likely would have yielded a niche not only in general thoracic surgery, but in cardiac as well.

So why did I keep working at the VA?

For one thing, despite my "epiphany" of 2006—and like nearly all of my part-time VA colleagues—I had grown accustomed to ignoring VA mediocrities. It became ingrained, a second nature.

Perhaps even more importantly, one should never underestimate "professional inertia," especially for busy academic doctors who already work extremely hard to keep up with a heavy clinical burden and the pressure of maintaining a cutting-edge research program on a par with full-time scientists. Both retooling a clinical practice and even simply moving a complex research facility (mine was located on the VA campus) couldn't just happen with the snap of a finger, and the thought of all that extra effort on top of what was already going on in my career had little appeal.

But there was more. At those times when I did consider my career options and questioned my longer-term goals, leaving the VA just didn't feel right. It didn't feel like the right thing to do. It felt like abandoning the vets. Vets who I increasingly felt deserved so much more than they were getting from the VA. With my departure, our aggressive program for surgical lung cancer care would likely come to a halt, or at least be slowed down significantly as it had for years before I signed on in 2003. I thought of the examples of Dallis and Marc, who had contributed their entire professional lives to the veterans, and I felt ashamed of my temptation to leave.

So by 2008, although I knew I was providing something important to my patients, I was beginning to accept that there was little I could do to make things work substantially better for the vets. I was beginning to comprehend not only that there was a system, a bureaucracy filled with inertia, but that many of the people who worked at the VA seemed to have a vested interest in resisting change. It was this combination of elements that, despite the widespread recognition of substandard care and the subsequent calls for quality improvement, made real change almost impossible to imagine. And yet, it was also at about this very time that I came to another, very different (and to me, much more startling) revelation.

Ever since I had first stepped foot on the Palo Alto VA campus to undertake a psychiatry rotation toward the end of medical school, I had viewed the vets as did everyone else at the VA: a downtrodden, unfortunate, and underprivileged class of people. People who perhaps had gotten few breaks, but who certainly had not made it far up the socioeconomic ladder of our society. Some, of course, were better off than others, but in general they did not have much. It therefore seemed a lucky break for them that the VA was there to make sure they had any healthcare at all. In any event, although perhaps deserving of our pity, there was never a general sense at the VA that these men and women were particularly deserving of our respect.

But then suddenly—perhaps because I had read something about the courage of our troops in the Middle East, perhaps for no reason at all—one day in 2008, I looked at the disheveled group of men and women sitting in the San Francisco VA clinic waiting room and I imagined all of them wearing their uniforms, standing at attention, well-trained and ready to go into battle, as each and every one of them most certainly had at one point or another in their lives. And then it really hit me: regardless of what had befallen each of these people, no matter what hardships they had endured and no matter what life had doled out to them, each and every one had made an enormous sacrifice for the benefit of his or her country. For the benefit of our security and our freedom. For the benefit of me, and of all of my colleagues. And every single one of them had made sacrifices that very few people in the course of "ordinary" life in our society are ever willing to make. Sacrifices that entailed, among other things, the willingness to risk their very lives. Regardless of how well we, as doctors, lived up to some Hippocratic ideal of respecting the humanity in all of our patients, whether at the comfortable clinics at UCSF or at the not-so-comfortable clinics at the county hospitals in San Francisco or San Jose, we did not need any excuses or Hippocratic oaths to respect the men and women sitting in the waiting area of the San Francisco VA. In a very profound way, each of them was a hero who had done something that we may not have had the courage to do ourselves.

This realization came way too late during my twenty-year association with the VA. It may seem surprising that it startled me and shook me up. And yet it powerfully contradicted every attitude toward the vets that I had encountered at the VA. Afterward, it was even harder for me to accept the inertial argument that "this was the VA."

And it was even harder for me to leave.

CHAPTER TEN

"Keep Your Head Low"

Despite a deepening commitment to the veterans, and despite my determination to make a difference for them, over time my early, somewhat naïve optimism waned. By the end of 2008, two of my initial reasons for optimism (Marc Marcotte and Dallis Manwaring) had both retired, exhausted by the grind against VA wheels. Tragically, not long after Dallis relinquished her daily battle on behalf of the vets, she succumbed to an even more personal battle with a cancer of her own.

By 2008, it had also become clearer to me how the machinery of the VA worked to prevent meaningful change. Certain elements of staff and committee meetings, for example, were no longer just a laughable reflection of our place within the federal bureaucracy. They were too often calculated components that held meaningful change in check—or even pushed it in the wrong direction. Bad patient outcomes, for example, were eschewed most aggressively if they contributed to bad statistics, and then they were eschewed at all costs, including the cost of a patient's right to choose a potentially lifesaving therapy, and sometimes the patients' right to hope.

The monthly staff meetings of our Surgical Service were a case in point. Mark Ratcliffe chaired these meetings, and by 2008 he used this forum to convey a repeated message: Risky patients were not to be brought to the OR. If there was significant chance that a patient might not survive at least thirty days past an operation, the operation should not be done.

✳ ✳ ✳

"Good morning everyone."

Mark Ratcliffe called one of our monthly Surgical Service meeting to order.

"Before we start with M&Ms, I want to focus people's attention on preoperative risk assessment. We're going to need to keep looking harder at those risks and make sure we're not bringing patients into the OR who have an unusually high chance of a bad outcome."

The M&Ms to which Ratcliffe was referring were not the world's best-selling candy, but a common abbreviation in American medicine for the discussion of morbidities (i.e., nonlethal complications) and mortalities (i.e., patient deaths). M&M conferences were one of the oldest traditions in modern medicine, the idealized intent being a forum designed to explore, openly and critically, a given group of doctors' bad outcomes. The hope was to grant the practitioners in that group a greater understanding of what had gone wrong and why, so that they could be better prepared to avoid similarly bad outcomes in the future. In the past, surgical M&Ms often deteriorated into a bloodbath of criticism and blame, but modern political correctness had taken most of the rough edges out of that tradition. Ratcliffe, it turned out, seemed to have an additional agenda altogether.

As the Surgical Service meeting progressed, the section chiefs for each subspecialty within the service were invited up to the podium one by one. Each ran through a list of their patients, identified by the first initials of their last names and the last four digits of their social security numbers, who had run into problems or who had died since the last service meeting. For each, brief descriptions of the case and the complication were presented, with a less detailed description of superficial wound infections and more detailed descriptions of any deaths.

"Did you classify that patient as high risk?" was Ratcliffe's first question to each chief immediately after the description of any death. The answer to this question was a double-edged hari-kari sword: if the patient was not high risk, then something must have gone very wrong to lead to the patient's demise. Strangely, that was the more acceptable scenario.

In his quest to reduce the number of surgical deaths at the San Francisco VA—a goal that I sensed even at that time was tied closely to the fact that the NSQIP program focused attention specifically on that component of a hospital's performance—Ratcliffe seemed convinced that his best method was to prevent any patient from going to the operating room if there was any serious chance that the patient might die.

That might seem to be a logical or even humane approach at first glance, but to doctors who had been trained to estimate risks and explain them carefully to their patients, this practice was simply a rationing of care that deprived certain patients of their inalienable right to informed consent—and to the right to fight for their own lives, their right to hope.

What my colleagues and I knew, sitting at those VA surgical staff meetings, was that the risk of doing nothing, of avoiding surgery altogether, could be at least as devastating as any potential complication. Patients realize this fact, as well. People don't just wander into an operating room; they sign on for *inevitable* pain and suffering precisely because they have something much more important to gain, and sometimes something much more terrifying to prevent. Patients have always been willing to risk a bad outcome, because without taking that risk something already wrong was going to get inevitably worse. The patients, we had been taught in medical school, were the only ones who had the right to assess the tradeoff between risk and potential reward from these procedures. Certainly not some VA bureaucrat.

Different section chiefs took different approaches to Mark Ratcliffe's inquisitions at Surgical Service meeting. Some would claim that there were hidden risks that could not have been appreciated pre-op. Although a clever evasion, these chiefs were opening themselves up to the threat of being lambasted for tolerating shoddy pre-op evaluations.

Other chiefs simply resorted instinctively to the true justification for having brought any patient to the operating room who had ever encountered a complication in the history of surgery itself: *complications happen.* That was why the revered principle of written informed consent had become so central in modern medical care. Not because doctors expect to make mistakes, but because risks can never be completely eliminated. Chances must always be taken in order for any patient to derive benefit. Patients must be informed of the risks if they are to make a fair decision about how much risk they are willing to take. Sometimes the risks are small; sometimes they are significant. But every surgeon at those Surgical Service meetings knew well that the only way to avoid surgical morbidities and mortalities entirely was *not to operate at all*. To nearly all of them, that was an inconceivable solution to the problem of the occasional bad outcome.

Mark presented the prohibition against risky surgeries starkly as a "Central VA policy." Even though I am sure no official memo to that effect ever crossed his desk, Mark seemed convinced that he was passing on what his own superiors had made clear to him: that surgical deaths were a blemish the VA could simply not afford. And therefore, VA surgeons could not afford them, either. Month after month he proclaimed to his largely part-time VA staff: regardless of how we managed our practices elsewhere, in this hospital we were VA employees—and so we had no choice but to comply with the policies the VA considered most prudent.

"Listen," Ratcliffe would often sum up at the end of our M&Ms, "the Central VA has simply decided that we do not bring high-risk patients to the operating room. It's just something we cannot do. We're part of the VA and so we have to follow VA policy. It's out of our hands."

Though I doubted Mark was quoting a truly written VA policy, I had no doubt that he was relating to us the message he believed his superiors had expressed to him about what Central VA expected. And yet those expectations were perplexing. I began to wonder what lay behind them. If the number of surgical deaths at the VA went down, who gained? If it was at the cost of many successfully lifesaving but "risky" operations, then the vets certainly did not gain. The gain was for the VA numbers. I began to wonder if this "policy" could be related to the miracle of NSQIP. By 2008, Mark had confided to me that NSQIP standing had become one of the single most important metrics by which each VA hospital, and the administrative leaders of each hospital, were being judged. What better way to improve NSQIP standing than to prevent any patient from reaching the operating room if there was a significant risk that the case might have a negative impact on the hospital's surgical statistics (or on the career advancement of its bureaucrats). The essence of NSQIP was numbers—the number of deaths or complications within thirty days following surgery. And we were ever increasingly exhorted not to perform risky surgeries. There had to be a connection.

Although I had not yet fully appreciated the profound role NSQIP had played in the careers of many top VA bureaucrats—possibly in salvaging the VA itself—I was already aware that every administrator involved in surgical matters at the VA paid a great deal of attention to NSQIP. The program was named National Surgical *Quality* Improvement, but what the program had truly succeeded in improving was VA national surgical *statistics*.

What was most perplexing about the increasingly emphatic warnings against "risky surgeries," however, was the very assumption, often true, that VA patients came to surgery in inherently worse condition than their non-VA counterparts. They were, therefore, inherently at higher risk for complications, including death. A prohibition against bringing "high-risk" patients to the VA operating room made no sense at all. In fact, to many of us at those staff meetings, the entire purpose of the VA was to provide a venue for high-risk care to the high-risk population of American veterans.

This perception of the VA's mission, however, may no longer have been shared by many of the individuals who had reached the upper echelons of both local and central VA administrations. Those people's careers were now judged not on the actual benefit derived by any given vet, but on the record of their performance as it was being calculated and tabulated by the VA. That meant that the statistics, and not the patients' lives, were the things that mattered most.

By 2008, Mark Ratcliffe had other problems to manage besides lowering surgical mortality statistics at his VA outpost.

Some of those problems related to the ambitions of some of the younger VA surgical recruits. One in particular, a newly minted, aggressive urologist, represented both the best and the worst of the VA. He was a talented surgeon with a strong commitment to his patients. But he was determined to become a leader in his field and fell prey to the VA attitude that saw vets as a resource to fulfill his dreams.

This young urologist was determined to become a national expert in the advanced use of surgical robots. Although urologists had already been using the complex, expensive technology to remove prostates, he wanted to prove that it would revolutionize other operations, too, such as the removal of a cancerous kidney. Of course, he didn't yet know how to perform such a procedure, but that was exactly where the VA patients came in handy. Even better, the San Francisco VA had already purchased a surgical robot for more than $1 million, and had found very little use for it. Mark supported the plan to use the San Francisco VA robot for this groundbreaking operation.

After months of searching for a patient, a complete robotic radical nephrectomy—possibly the first of its kind in VA history—was scheduled at the San Francisco VA. The procedure would have been straightforward through a conventional incision, or possibly even with a non-robotic yet minimally invasive approach. Not having been present, I cannot say how the prospect of being the first veteran in San Francisco to undergo this very difficult and complex version of an otherwise straightforward operation was described to the patient who ended up signing the informed consent form. There were no documented benefits for this unconventional approach, and the risks were largely unknown.

And not having been present for the operation, I don't know exactly what happened during the case, either. What I do know is that things progressed very slowly as the operative team felt its way through unfamiliar waters. Eventually, the approach and the use of the robot led to a massive tear in the patient's aorta, the blood vessel that carries blood from the heart to the rest of the body.

The patient bled to death before steps could be taken to save his life.

In addition to fallout from surgical misadventures, Mark was faced with direct, frontal attacks. Another up-and-coming general surgeon decided to advance her own career by undermining Mark's position as the surgical chief in San Francisco so that she could be anointed in Mark's place. She turned her abundant charm on the hospital's chief of staff, Diana Nicoll.

One morning I received an unusually subdued phone call from Mark about this mutinous surgeon. "She has already convinced Diana Nicoll that I am an incompetent leader," Mark told me. "She's out of control. If I let her continue, she's going to destroy my reputation. The only way to stop her is to fire her. So that's what I have to do. When that happens, I know she'll go ballistic, and then she'll probably go to the press. To spare us all that heartache, after I fire her, I'm going to resign."

Floored by this unexpected revelation, I kept my composure long enough to convince Mark to reconsider his plan . . . and to let me try to broker a peace between the two of them that might prevent their mutual destruction. To my immense surprise, they both took me up on my offer, and, even more surprisingly, I convinced them to coexist.

Through it all, I got a glimpse of the immense pressure Mark felt to be many things to many people at the VA. In particular, I could understand better his apparent drive to please his superiors and provide the type of surgical statistics and NSQIP performance they seemed so much to want.

∗ ∗ ∗

During my tenure there, another ambitious young surgeon began to build his career at the San Francisco VA in the field of vascular surgery. At that time, repair of the aorta in the abdomen was already being performed routinely through another kind of "minimally invasive" approach, one that depended on large tubes (or "catheters") that could be threaded inside a patient's blood vessels. This particular vascular surgeon, however, was determined to become a local expert at catheter-based repair of the aorta just as it exited the patient's heart inside the chest. That meant he would have to train for several months far from the San Francisco VA, and Mark Ratcliffe demanded that he find a temporary replacement surgeon before he left.

Though few surgeons were amenable to picking up these duties for such a short time, he eventually found an elderly, retired surgeon who was willing to come to San Francisco. Mark insisted that this older surgeon complete at least one successful major vascular surgery at our VA before the young buck left town, and that the younger surgeon proctor his older colleague and be present in the operating room throughout the case.

A routine, conventional repair of a patient's aorta was hastily scheduled, but the young surgeon boldly decided to let the "new guy" perform the case without his own involvement.

The operation went very wrong. It took a lot longer than most, and in the end the patient ended up hemorrhaging when the aortic reconstruction began to fall apart. Finally, the young, San Francisco VA vascular surgeon realized that he had to join the operation; but by the time he did, and despite his obviously higher surgical skills, there was nothing he or anyone else could do to stop the patient from bleeding to death on the operating table.

✳ ✳ ✳

The San Francisco VA Research and Development Committee (of which I was a member) reviewed the case of this vascular surgery debacle—not because the operation turned out tragically for the patient, but because it had also involved a human research protocol violation that was unrelated to the patient's death. In addition to deciding not to act as a proctor in the case as he had agreed, the young surgeon had also decided to go ahead and enroll the patient in an experimental program, called a "clinical trial," that involved administration of a new drug that was still under study. The problem was that the research protocol insisted that patients only be enrolled in the trial if he was the operative surgeon.

This young surgeon, Dr. Carter, it turned out, had also been accused of routinely practicing several other types of relatively minor human research deviations. None of these other missteps had had anything like the impact on patient care of his delegation of surgical responsibility in the particularly unfortunate case of the unproctored operation. But a regularly demonstrated disregard for understandably sacrosanct regulations, those implemented to allow close oversight of human research, was a potentially serious matter.

Most people, in fact, would have viewed most of what Carter had done wrong as relatively innocuous. The majority of the transgressions had to do with patients' consents for the use of their discarded tissues for research purposes after their operations were over. Surgeons traditionally viewed tissues removed from their patients—tissues that would otherwise end up either burned as medical waste or preserved in wax and stored in pathology archives for decades—as freely available to those who hoped to use them to advance medical knowledge. In the modern era, however, ethics committees and institutional review boards (powerful committees known as "IRBs") had made it clear that researchers needed patients' express permissions to use anything that had come out of their bodies. Exceptions were made for tissues that had already been archived in years past and for which it would be prohibitively difficult to track down patients for their consent. For all new specimens, however, the living, breathing patients needed to be consented before any of their tissues would be allowed to leave the operating room for a research lab. And that meant that each patient needed to be consented prior to surgery. No written consent, no specimen. The rules had become pretty cut and dried.

Actually bothering to bring a consent form to a patient, bothering to explain the research goals, methods, and potential risks, and bothering to answer any lingering questions all took time and energy. For something that "couldn't possibly hurt the patient," it must have all seemed a bit unnecessary to someone like this young Dr. Carter. Especially at the VA. Some of his patients were therefore consented after their surgeries, as they were recovering either in the ICU or on the regular wards. That was a protocol violation. But for some patients, he had simply forged their signatures, in some cases many months after the fact, claiming later that he had consented the patients orally before surgery. This practice came to light when a medical student realized what was going on and was advised by a faculty member in whom she confided to go to the San Francisco VA's research compliance officer.

And so an investigation was initiated and a file was compiled. I heard about the whole mess from Mark Ratcliffe, who was very concerned that the affair would threaten Carter's career. Human research violations had become a serious issue in academic medicine. Part of the issue was that even small violations, if done intentionally, reflected a lapse in judgment and a lapse in respect for rules that had been created to protect patient rights.

On top of the missing and falsified patient consents, Carter had also committed another notable VA offense: he had handed out to the same student his password to the VA's massive computerized medical record and electronic medical ordering system. Cyber security had become an obsession at the VA ever since the theft of an unencrypted laptop and hard drive from a VA data analyst in May 2006 had resulted in the potential compromise of social security numbers and other personal information on 26.5 million veterans. Cyber security lapses had become unconditionally unacceptable. When these transgressions were lumped together with the possibly unnecessary death of a patient whose operation had been conducted in yet another violation of a research protocol, a pattern of disregard for human research regulations could very well have triggered harsh discipline from the VA R&D Committee. Mark was concerned that Carter could face the revocation of research privileges that might make his continued academic appointment at UCSF untenable.

The R&D Committee at the San Francisco VA was an interesting beast. When Mark Ratcliffe first appointed me to the committee, I had not expected a research body to wield much power or influence. But this particular VA outpost prided itself on its widely respected research program, which was bolstered largely through its very close ties with UCSF. A constant shortage of space at the university led many leading faculty members to conduct some or all of their studies on the VA campus. Eventually, that meant that tens of millions of research dollars, mostly from the federal government's National Institutes of Health, were flowing through the institution, more research dollars than at any other VA site. And for this reason, the R&D Committee was taken seriously by the powers that be.

Attendance at the R&D Committee meeting the day that Carter's case was reviewed was unusually heavy. What surprised me, though, was the presence of someone who was not even a member of the committee: Hospital Chief of Staff Diana Nicoll. Nicoll had participated only in one or two of these meetings during the four or five years of my regular attendance. As the meeting wound its way through a lot of relatively boring material, Nicoll sat patiently, occasionally uttering an "Oh, that sounds like an interesting study" or an "I will be very interested to see what they find" as we reviewed new research protocols that were up for approval.

Toward the end of the meeting, the research compliance officer finally presented Carter's case to the committee. At first, only the problems with written informed consent were described.

"So, allow me to try to crystallize what you've told us," the committee chairman chimed in at a lull in the presentation. "According to Dr. Carter, the patients were appropriately introduced to the study before their operations, but they didn't actually sign the consent form until after their operations. So that means that when the specimens were collected from the operating room, the patients had not yet signed informed consent."

"That's right."

"And that, I assume," the chairman continued, "is inconsistent with the protocol as approved by the IRB, which I assume has the standard stipulation that patients be consented prior to the collection of tissue specimens."

"Can I ask," one of the other committee members interjected, "were the specimens first sent to the pathology lab, and then only later brought to Dr. Carter's lab for analysis? In that case, maybe the consent was signed before the tissues were actually 'collected.'"

"Yes, exactly," Diana Nicoll's animated voice suddenly punctuated the discussion. "Are we even sure that any specimens reached Dr. Carter's lab before the consents were signed?"

"Uh, actually," the research compliance officer responded, "we do know that the specimens went straight from the operating room to Dr. Carter's research lab because that was one of the student's roles, to go to the operating room during the operation and bring the specimen back to the lab."

The expression on Diana Nicoll's face immediately sank, reflecting her distinct displeasure with this response. Although the purpose of her attendance at this particular R&D Committee meeting seemed finally to be emerging, it was still unclear why she seemed determined to weigh in on Dr. Carter's behalf.

"During your interviews," the chairman picked up on the uncomfortable pause in the proceedings, demonstrating his own determination to move things along, "were you able to ascertain whether Dr. Carter appreciated the need for written informed consent prior to the collection of human tissue specimens?"

"Yes," the compliance officer answered, "he did. And in our discussions we identified several critical structural factors that contributed to the root cause of these delayed consents."

"Dr. Carter is a very level-headed person," Diana Nicoll again jumped in. "I'm sure he understands the importance of the consent process, and it's not too surprising that there were mitigating factors."

After a brief discussion of the mitigating factors that made it inconvenient to find appropriate consent forms at the appropriate times, the committee chairman seemed ready to wrap things up.

"And so what do you propose as the disposition for this case. Shall we notify the IRB? And what about Dr. Carter's lack of protocol compliance."

"Yes," the compliance officer said, also seeming relieved to be reaching the end of this review, "we should notify the IRB about this protocol deviation, but indicate that our assessment is that there was no risk to patients as a result. In addition to the structural changes we discussed, Dr. Carter has already agreed to repeat his human research subject training and certification. In fact, I think he has already completed that online."

With the VA rumor mill as efficient as it was, I was sure that I was not the only one in the room who had heard not only about the missing consents, but also about the forged consents. And what, I asked myself, about the cyber security breach? I knew that the next thing that would happen would be a motion for the committee to accept the suggested disposition, and then for the committee to vote.

"I move that this committee resolves to accept the suggested disposition." The words emanated from somewhere around the teak table.

"I second the motion."

The reality was that I, too, did not consider the omitted consent forms to be a truly serious ethical breach. And if a bigger deal than necessary was being made about the missing signatures, I could even understand why Carter had thought it okay in the grand scheme of things to go ahead and complete the forms with his own hand. Since Carter had clearly worked with the medical student in question and had developed a trust in the young woman's judgment, one could even comprehend why he had, in a moment of eagerness to enlist assistance in the collection of clinical data, taken the unnecessarily risky step of giving the student his own password to the heavily guarded VA electronic medical record and ordering system.

But the reality also was that Carter just did not seem to care about the rules. And even though it was not the inappropriate participation in a research protocol that had led to the intraoperative demise of one of his recent patients, the protocol violation in that case happened to have been his not doing the operation himself—and that might have, in fact, been a significant contributing factor in the tragic outcome.

"Before we vote," I raised my voice instinctively, catching people's attention before the chairman had a chance to call for a show of hands. "Um, before we vote," I continued in a more reasonable tone of voice, "weren't there a couple of other issues to be discussed?"

If a pink elephant had suddenly crashed onto the teak wood of the conference table, there could not have been a more profound wave of astonishment than the one that made its way around the room.

"I understand," I continued, "that Dr. Carter had to get some of these consents over the phone, even after the patients had gone home from the hospital, and that in those cases he signed the patients' names himself and backdated the forms to the times that the surgeries took place."

"Dr. Mann." I was not terribly surprised to find Diana Nicoll responding to me herself. "Are you quite sure that is what happened?"

"Actually . . ." The compliance officer stepped up. "Dr. Carter did tell us that he did have to call some patients and that he asked them if it was all right for him to sign their names on the consent forms. Unfortunately, he had not indicated on the forms that that's what he had done."

"And does Dr. Carter now understand," the R&D Committee chairman asked, "that these activities were all outside the bounds of Good Clinical Practice and are not considered acceptable research informed consent?"

Good Clinical Practice is an international standard for human research published by a body known as the International Council on Harmonisation. It is considered a sacrosanct guide to the conduct of research involving human subjects.

"Yes, he does."

"Well, these irregularities," the chairman concluded, "are a little more substantive than what we had just heard. Perhaps we need to make sure Dr. Carter is proctored during his next five or ten research consents so that he can feel confident that he's getting things right and so that this committee can reach closure on these issues."

"And what about the patient," a new voice emerged suddenly from the corner of the room, apparently emboldened by what had just transpired, "who died after Dr. Carter delegated an unapproved investigator to perform a study operation in his place? That seems like a more serious type of violation."

Nicoll's demeanor went from bad to worse.

"Well, actually," the compliance officer began, now seeing an opportunity to quell the storm, "we did review that case carefully with Dr. Ratcliffe, and he confirmed that the complication was simply a risk of the operation itself, and was not in any way related to the patient's participation in that study."

"Well, then" the chairman said decisively, "let me propose an alternative resolution: Dr. Carter shall be put on a period of probation with regard to patient enrollment in his clinical studies. During that time, he will be proctored with regard to written informed consent until which time that he has completed ten consecutive successful consents with no protocol or GCP violations. During this period, his studies can remain open for enrollment."

"That sounds very fair," Diana Nicoll proclaimed. "Strict, but fair."

Quickly someone moved for the committee to adopt the resolution, and just as quickly someone else seconded the move. This time, a vote was called that yielded near unanimous adoption by the committee. A few people didn't vote. Carter had avoided a research suspension, or any truly serious consequences at all.

"Before we completely wrap up the discussion," this time I spoke more out of curiosity than out of any sense of oversight duty, "wasn't there also a problem with Dr. Carter giving out his VistA username and password to the student who came forward?"

A slight shudder ran through the room. Everyone understood the seriousness of a cyber security violation at the VA. No one had any idea how to react.

Except for Diana Nicoll.

"Oh, yes, that was such a silly thing to do." Nicoll's voice was as calm and steady as if someone had asked her for the time of day. "Don't worry. That is of no concern to this committee. The matter's already been discussed with our local cyber security officer, and the whole thing is clearly in their purview. They'll be tying up any loose ends."

And with that, the chairman did not hesitate to adjourn the meeting.

Nicoll's presence had been imposing, and so, clearly, was her influence over the committee; the surgeon was let off with a slap on the wrist.

I never understood why he had Nicoll's protection. But the protection was real, powerful, and unmistakable. And so, too, I learned, was Diana Nicoll's influence over the staff of the San Francisco VA.

* * *

One day toward the end of August 2009, on the eve of his departure from San Francisco for a meeting at the NIH in Bethesda, Maryland, Mark Ratcliffe called me into his office. After we were seated in his facing armchairs, his mood turned strangely somber and he looked me straight in the eye.

"Michael," he said, leaning closer to ensure I focused on his words, "I want you to listen to me. I want you to keep your head low. Do you understand what I mean? Very serious people out there are gunning for you, so you need to watch yourself."

His words came so out of the blue that I didn't know how to react . . . or what to say. People were gunning for me? Who? How? Why? Although I had certainly annoyed a few people over the years, nothing I'd done seemed to me to justify such a serious threat. I listened intently to his next words.

"You can't afford any complications right now; you need to cool your jets. Do you hear me? Do you understand what I'm trying to say? I don't want you to take on any risky or dangerous cases—at least not until I get back."

Something in his manner, probably his visible anxiety, reminded me of his own professional "near-death" experience. This was no longer the exuberant mentor, friend, and confidant who had labored with excitement to recruit me into his academic Mecca. And though I had had almost nothing to do with Dr. Nicoll throughout my six years on her staff, I also recalled the power she had effortlessly displayed at one of our R&D Committee meetings. If "serious people" were gunning for me, she could very well have been one of them.

I still didn't understand how to grapple with Mark's warning. It seemed bizarre. But it was worrisome enough to take seriously, and I made an honest promise to "cool my jets" until his return.

CHAPTER ELEVEN

A VA Land Mine

For 24 years, Navy Cmdr. Jeff Hawker served his country, leaving active duty to continue treating his military brethren as a Department of Veterans Affairs doctor. After he started working at the Salem [Virginia] VA Medical Center, though, he said it took just a few months for officials at the medical center to oust him and to destroy his career after he reported dangerous medical practices. . . . Hawker said he was the victim of a so-called "sham peer review," a problem many say is widespread in the VA and little reported because the victims fear bringing attention to their negative reviews. Hawker said vindictive local VA officials have effectively ended his career after he voiced serious concerns about patient safety at a busy Virginia hospital, including a doctor performing procedures Hawker said he wasn't trained to do and life-threatening medical errors. Worse, Hawker said, veterans there are still

at serious risk months after he reported
the problems.

—Stars and Stripes [19]

When Mark Ratcliffe warned me to "keep my head low" on August 27, 2009, I had no idea that VA doctors and their careers were being targeted at VA facilities around the country in response to "disruptive behavior." I had never been involved in disciplinary actions during my twenty years in the profession. And although I knew I was constantly pushing the San Francisco VA to attempt a higher level of care in thoracic surgery than would otherwise have been expected (closer to the level we achieved at the university), I didn't consider myself to be "disruptive." I did not yet have access to closely held national VA data that would later explain why my brand of aggressive thoracic surgery was anathema to local VA administrators, and a threat to their annual bonuses. But less than twenty-four hours after Mark's strange warning, I stepped on a VA land mine that eventually brought an end to advanced, high-risk thoracic surgery at the San Francisco VA.

One of the achievements we had made in thoracic surgery at the San Francisco VA during my tenure was the introduction of a "minimally invasive" form of lung cancer surgery known as "VATS[20] lobectomy." Although the cure rates had never been proven to be any different with this approach, the small incisions and minimal disruption of the chest wall made our patients' recoveries easier and faster. The technique also promised to make more definitive lung cancer treatments accessible to a larger number of veterans with other significant, limiting medical problems, including better tolerance of a complete course of postoperative chemotherapy when necessary.

---

[19] Heath Druzin, "Doctor Says 'Sham Peer Review' Used to Destroy His Career After Pointing Out VA Problems," Stars and Stripes, December 15, 2014, accessed January 25, 2015, http://www.stripes.com/news/veterans/doctor-says-sham-peer-review-used-to-destroy-his-career-after-pointing-out-va-problems-1.319484.

[20] Video-assisted thoracoscopic surgery

On the morning of August 28, 2009, I participated in a symposium in San Francisco featuring national experts in VATS lobectomy techniques, hoping to further improve and expand the success of our program. My attendance was enabled, in part, by one of my colleagues' routine assignment to cover any emergencies that might arise among cardiothoracic patients at the VA. It was part of a "community call" approach advocated by Mark Ratcliffe. He wanted to avoid any delay or confusion when urgent needs arose, knowing that, as part-time VA physicians and as academic doctors, any member of his staff could be otherwise engaged at any given moment when an emergency unfolded. The attending who was on call for any given day needed to stay available, needed to be familiar with all cardiac patients in the hospital, and was responsible for taking care of all urgent or emergent problems that arose outside of the usual schedule, no matter who might have treated the patient in question in the past.

I decided to leave the VATS lobectomy conference early, however, when I received an odd phone call from my colleague on call. It seemed that a patient whose aortic valve I had replaced about a month or so prior had come back to the hospital in the middle of the night before, complaining of shortness of breath. A chest X-ray revealed fluid around the lung, and he had been admitted for observation and treatment. In the morning, however, an echocardiogram was obtained that indicated another fluid buildup, this time around the heart itself. This second fluid collection, known as a pericardial effusion, was more dangerous, since in a tight space surrounded by a tough, fibrous sac, it could put pressure on the patient's heart and impede its ability to pump blood to the body. The patient had not yet reached that life-threatening condition called "tamponade," but unchecked it was a distinct possibility that needed to be averted. Luckily, a fairly simple operation through a very small incision that required about fifteen minutes of operating room time could solve the problem.

My colleague was on call that day. It was certainly a reasonable and courteous thing for him to call and let me know about a patient on whom I had recently operated. In fact, it would have been even better if I had gotten the call the night before. I asked when the OR would have the time available to get this short but important case done. He told me it would probably be sometime in the afternoon.

"I'm at a VATS lobectomy symposium right now across town, and I have a packed clinic over at UCSF starting at one," I told my counterpart who was at the VA. "I wonder if you might be able to do the case when they're ready?" It was actually his responsibility to get the case done, but my somewhat deferential response reflected my own desire to continue to manage this patient's surgical treatment, never having fully bought into the concept of relinquishing this responsibility as part of our "community call" approach.

On the other hand, I knew that a lot of cancer patients would be waiting for me at UCSF. Many of them had desperate problems, and had been referred to me for surgical care that doctors in the community were not comfortable providing. As was often the case for people in our field, I was torn by conflicting but equally compelling patient needs. Whereas my colleague had been assigned specifically to serve as my substitute at the VA, where he could provide essentially identical care, there was no one who could take on the mantel of what I needed to accomplish in my clinic at UCSF.

"I can talk to the OR and see if they'll let you do it after five." My colleague's response was not what I had expected. The implication had been that the case was somewhat urgent, and he was on call specifically to manage this type of situation.

"Maybe it would be better if you could get the case done sooner," I said. "Besides, my clinics often run late and you know how the OR can be about trying to get cases done late in the day, especially on a Friday." I had been confused by my colleague's response, but I was running through priorities myself as much as I was trying to convince him to help out.

"That's okay. The patient's very comfortable now, and they're not seeing any tamponade physiology. It should be fine."

"Hmm. Can cardiology simply put in a drain right now, so that we have at least temporary control and don't need to worry about any sudden decompensation?"

"I talked to the cardiologists who read the echo, and they said that they can't reach it with a needle." That was unfortunate.

"I think it's a bit dangerous to hope that nothing changes and that the OR doesn't get tied up when they're down to a skeleton crew after five," I concluded. "Is there a reason you wouldn't be able to get the case done as soon as they're ready in the early afternoon?"

"I'll talk to the OR." There was a long, uncomfortable pause as I wondered exactly what he would discuss with the OR administrators.

"So, you'll do the case?" I finally broke the silence.

"Why don't we see how things go," he responded cryptically. "I think it might be fine to schedule things for after five."

There was another uncomfortable silence. I had asked my colleague three times if he would follow protocol and take care of a simple but potentially lifesaving procedure. I had not really understood any of the answers, or what he was trying to tell me.

"Okay, thanks." After another uncomfortable silence, we both hung up our phones.

I was confused, but the bottom line was that I had lost all confidence in letting him take care of the situation. Within another couple of seconds, I had decided to leave the symposium early and to head over to the VA before going to my clinic at UCSF. I called the clinic nurses and told them to apologize to my patients and explain an emergency had come up and that I wouldn't be able to make it over until two p.m. I then called the VA OR, who told me that they had heard about the case, that they did have an open room, and that a cardiac anesthesiologist was available to handle the operation. I then spoke to my colleague on call one more time. He was in his VA office, and I let him know that I had rearranged my day and was coming to the hospital and hoped to get the case done. By then it was about noon, and two hours should have been enough time to get everything done and for me to get over to the UCSF clinic. This time, I simply asked my colleague if he would be available to take over for me at two p.m., just in case there were more delays. To this he readily agreed.

Once at the hospital, I reviewed the situation carefully with the entire OR team, including the cardiac anesthesiologist and our nurse, Michael Baker. Although the patient was very stable lying on his gurney in the pre-op holding area, his condition carried the risk of a sudden, potentially life-threatening drop in blood pressure with the administration of general anesthesia. We therefore agreed to the very unusual step of making sure that not only would I be in the room when the patient went to sleep, but that the patient would be already prepped for surgery and that I would be in full surgical gown and gloves, ready to make an immediate incision if necessary as soon as the anesthesia medicine hit. Although it was not yet one p.m., and although the anesthesiologist assured me that everything was ready to go, I confirmed that everyone understood my need to head over to UCSF at two p.m., and knew that my colleague was fully informed and standing by to take over, just in case.

But this was the VA, and even a relatively urgent case, one that could have been teed up in an efficient OR within ten or fifteen minutes, took over an hour to prepare. I had waited in my office for word from the team, but when none came, I called in shortly after two. When I was told they were *almost* ready to start, I indicated that I'd have my colleague come right over to the OR in my place, according to plan. I called him, and he agreed to head right down the hall. I made my way to UCSF.

Even for the VA, it later struck me as very odd that the anesthesiologist went ahead and administered anesthesia in the several minutes it took my colleague to walk down the hall, without once asking for me to be called and without ever making sure, as he had promised, that either I or another cardiac surgery attending was not only in the room, but fully outfitted and ready to go. As bad luck would have it, the patient did have a negative reaction to anesthesia. But having followed through with all the other preparations, my chief cardiac resident, himself a fully trained general surgeon, was scrubbed at the patient's side, and within a minute or so had completed the lifesaving maneuver himself, albeit without the supervision of an attending cardiac surgeon.

Despite everything I knew about the VA, I was also surprised that this particular anesthesiologist went to Diana Nicoll's office immediately after the case, telling her that I had recklessly abandoned my patient and had nearly caused his death. When I responded to Nicoll's page, I was even more surprised at how difficult it was for her to understand that, although I was very upset to hear what had happened, despite all of our careful discussion and planning, I had conscientiously tried to put a mechanism in place for the safe and effective management of the patient's case, albeit one that depended on the anesthesiologist's attention and cooperation.

Nicoll didn't want to hear what I had to say. According to what the anesthesiologist had told her, a patient had almost died and I was to blame. That was the last word. Her judgmental attitude left me baffled.

Soon after, Nicoll formed a "comprehensive review committee" to investigate this case, as well as a pair of high-risk cases of mine in which the patients had died postoperatively . . . the committee was told to look into "additional cases" if it thought that they might uncover deficiencies in my practice at the VA. By then, my "on-call" surgical colleague had corroborated my explanation for what had happened on August 28, and even the anesthesiologist had admitted that there was no reason for his overly hasty administration of anesthesia. Independent quality assurance bodies had already carefully analyzed the care that my team and I had delivered in the cases of post-surgical death, and had found our performances to be error-free. So I approached this investigation naïvely confident that my responsibility was simply to relate the truth. I had no conception at the time of hospital bylaws, potential disciplinary actions against physicians, or what harm this "comprehensive review committee" might have been capable of inflicting. It all seemed like an appeasement of the anesthesiologist, who seemed from the beginning to want to deflect criticism for what he had done.

Brian Cason, chief of the Anesthesia Service and a good friend of my accuser, was assigned to chair the committee; a cardiologist and an ophthalmologist were appointed from the San Francisco VA staff, but Ratcliffe took the unusual step of bringing in a fourth member from outside San Francisco, a New York VA cardiac surgeon for whom we both had great respect. Mark indicated that he thought this outside participant would give the committee additional credibility; in retrospect, I wondered if Mark had been trying to lend me some unstated support.

During my interview before the committee, this outside VA surgeon was the only one who seemed determined to understand the facts of my case. He listened carefully to my detailed descriptions of the care that had been provided in the high-risk thoracic cases, and he seemed perturbed by the anesthesiologist's behavior in the cardiac case. Cason, on the other hand, clearly assumed I was at fault, while the two others remained relatively silent. Meanwhile, I had decided to go ahead with plans for a family leave of absence from my heavy duties at the VA so I could help care for a member of my family who had fallen seriously ill, a leave that had the added benefit of defusing tension at the hospital during the committee's investigation.

The committee met in October and November, but I didn't hear the results until January. In an unrelated meeting that month with Nancy Ascher about my work at UCSF (which had continued uninterrupted during my leave from the VA), she offhandedly asked if I had seen the committee's report. I hadn't.

"Apparently, you've been completed vindicated."

Although Nancy related this development in her normal, nonchalant manner, the news actually came as a surprise to me. I had no idea what might have happened had the opposite outcome materialized, but I was just as pleased not to be finding out. The management of complex, difficult cases almost always involves judgment calls and decisions that yield no absolute rights and wrongs. And when these produce an unfortunate outcome, Monday-morning quarterbacking abounds. If this committee truly had been given license to dig into my most difficult and problematic cases at the VA and had not come up with a single substantial criticism of my work, I couldn't imagine a stronger endorsement.

It was February, though, before I saw the committee's report myself. Mark Ratcliffe finally sat me down in his office to give me the news of my exoneration.

"Basically," Mark began, somewhat hesitantly, "the committee decided that you hadn't done anything wrong." He seemed unsure how best to describe to me what was written in the committee's report, which apparently had been available since December fifteenth. He appeared reluctant to encourage me—or worse yet, to embolden me—but the truth seemed to be that there was very little that could be described as damning in the report.

"Nothing?" I was a little incredulous that this proceeding could possibly have left me completely in the clear. "You mean they couldn't find one thing in any of those cases to suggest I had made any mistakes at all?"

"Well," Mark responded, "after interviewing a lot of people, they did call into question whether the hospital has been providing adequate support for thoracic surgery, and they recommended that more resources be made available to you." Among other things, it was suggested that my program be provided the benefit of dedicated nursing and of at least one more part-time thoracic surgeon.

"Unbelievable" was the only response that came to my mind. With the participation of an objective outsider, this committee had apparently been forced to take a relatively honest look at what was going on and reported back that thoracic surgery at the San Francisco VA was deserving of greater support.

"Can I have a copy of the report?"

"I will see if I can get one for you." Now that, I thought, was more typical of the VA. Needing to jump through hoops to make a formal report on my own work available for me to read.

"All right," I went on. "Well at least it sounds like this is all behind us."

"Not exactly," Mark answered, knowing that the unpleasant part of this discussion was about to unfold. "We're asking you to be proctored during your next five cases, and we're instituting certain rules that you'll need to follow."

"What?" Although I had anticipated some sort of unjustified censure from this investigation, I didn't expect the VA to ignore the formal findings of the committee and to come up instead with some completely arbitrary demand. "Was that the recommendation of the comprehensive review?"

"No," Mark readily admitted. "They only recommended that you get more resources."

"And they didn't find any deficiencies in my care, and no lapses in my professionalism?"

"No," Mark answered again, very matter-of-factly.

"Then how can you justify this 'proctoring'? And why should I agree?" It then occurred to me to ask, "Who is this 'we,' anyway?"

"Diana Nicoll," Mark answered only this last and simplest of my questions, "Brian Cason, and myself. Look," he continued, "there really is no room for discussion here, Michael. The feelings regarding this are very strong."

"Feelings?" I knew it would be better for me to keep my cool. "Whose feelings?" I repeated in a quieter tone. "What about due process? What about some respect for what we're trying to do?"

"Michael," Mark said, now also straining to maintain his demeanor, "I really need you to listen to me. There are very serious people out there and you need to watch yourself. Just listen to me, otherwise there's nothing I can do to help."

The scene was now reminiscent of Mark's "Keep your head low" warning on the eve of the entire affair that had triggered this "comprehensive review."

"Okay, but give me one good reason why I should agree to this proctoring."

"Because I'm the chief of this service, Michael," Mark replied, "and because sometimes I make unreasonable requests."

Since acceptance of the proctoring would be taken as an implicit confession of guilt, I was initially inclined to reject the idea as an unreasonable form of harassment. However, Ratcliffe from the VA, along with David Jablons and Scott Merrick from UCSF, all urged me to accept it and the message it would send to the VA rumor mill about the result of the investigation. "It'll all blow over," they told me, "and the VA gossip will soon move on to a juicier story."

In the end, my only other real choice was to leave the VA entirely. There was certainly some temptation finally to do so, although my successful lab program was still rooted at the VA campus, and it would still have been inconvenient to suddenly reshape my appointment to full-time UCSF. But more importantly, I simply could not ignore what my departure would mean, at least in the near term, for the care of the veterans who were showing up in San Francisco with lung cancer and other thoracic surgical problems. Although two UCSF surgeons had been asked to step in, little or no serious thoracic surgery was getting done at the San Francisco VA during my leave of absence—just as thoracic surgery had languished at this VA hospital for at least two years before my appointment in 2003. If I did leave, I would be abandoning too many weary and terrified faces, too many underserved heroes, primarily because of an implicit slight to my local reputation.

And so I agreed to the proctoring, and to the special rules.

Ratcliffe "suggested" that I meet with Cason prior to formally resuming my clinical work at the VA. I brought David Jablons, who was assigned to be my proctor for the five cases, to the tête-à-tête. Cason told me, among other things, that one more surgical death would mean the end of my career at the VA.

It was a remarkable threat. I couldn't help but conclude that it wasn't my competence or incompetence as a surgeon that had bothered Cason, Nicoll, and even Ratcliffe. It was the surgical mortalities themselves. It was the numbers. Perhaps it was the increasing emphasis placed on the hospital's NSQIP ranking, which, Ratcliffe had confided some time before, had been dropping precipitously. And which likely had negatively impacted the annual bonuses of Nicoll, Ratcliffe, and Cason, who were the chief of staff, the chief of surgery, and the chief of anesthesia of our hospital.

It had been true, I realized then, that much of the fuss about thoracic surgery had revolved around the surgical mortalities. Even though there had been no mistakes identified that had led to any of the deaths on our service, and even though these patients each had died in pursuit of a risky but real hope to be saved from an otherwise certain cancer death, the administration of our hospital could not seem to let them go.

David and I pointed out to Brian Cason that the only way to ensure the absence of any surgical deaths was not to do any thoracic surgery at all, hardly an acceptable approach. Cason was unmoved.

But there was another way: For the next year, I reluctantly abandoned my customary approach to managing the service and obeyed Ratcliffe's directives to avoid operating on "risky" patients. Uncharacteristically, I began saying "no" to a lot of cases at Multi-Disciplinary Chest Conference. There were no postoperative deaths among my patients that year, and not even one obvious complication.

That's not to say that none of the VA patients got into any trouble within their chests. One day, for example, I was asked by my resident if I had seen the recent chest X-rays of one of the nonsurgical patients in the ICU. I had not, and the resident promptly asked me to take a look.

The veteran had been struggling in the ICU for some time. He was too sick to eat, and the ICU team that was managing him had been justifiably anxious to start delivering nutrition into the patient's intestines. Without a source of calories and protein, the patient would consume his own tissues in an effort to generate the energy necessary to attempt a recovery from his severe illness. In doing so, he would grow even weaker in a deadly downward spiral. A decision was made to place a feeding tube through the patient's nose that would go down into his stomach or intestines.

One of the first things a good medical student learns is not to force a piece of medical paraphernalia that is not going smoothly into whatever part of the body it needs to go. The second critical lesson is to assess the success of any "placement" procedure with objective evidence confirming that the device has gone correctly to where it needed to be before initiating its use—especially if misplacement could make that use potentially disastrous.

I was told that a resident had placed this particular veteran's feeding tube late at night, hoping to conform to his team's directive to get the feeding process started by the next morning's rounds. Unsupervised, the resident pushed the tube into the patient's nose, hoping it would make the correct ninety-degree turn down into the patient's esophagus and stomach, and kept pushing until it would go no more.

At that point, in accordance with standard safety procedures, the resident ordered a chest X-ray to confirm proper placement. The resident did actually look at the chest X-ray that he or she had ordered, did notice that the tube in this case had not seemed to progress all the way into the patient's stomach, and did therefore return to the patient's bedside to push it down even farther into the patient's body.

What was apparent to me as my own resident pulled up this patient's X-ray films, now several days later, was that the initial film clearly revealed that the tube must have missed the opening in the patient's esophagus, or "food pipe," altogether, and had entered instead the opening of his trachea, or "windpipe." My resident and I could see the end of the tube sitting in his lung. I incredulously asked if the tube had not been removed from the lung; the answer was abundantly clear in successive chest X-rays from the following days that my resident silently pulled up from the computer. There was a steady build up of fluid over the course of those days, fluid that began taking up space that should have been available for the veteran's struggling lungs. The last film in the series showed a left chest completely filled with fluid, in a patient, whom I was told, not surprisingly, lost the ability to extract an adequate amount of oxygen from the air, and who then succumbed to a cardiac arrest.

Part of the subsequent attempts at the patient's emergent resuscitation was the placement of a much larger tube directly through the chest wall, a tube that drained liters of thick, frothy, infected feeding solution from the patient's chest. Feeding solution that everyone on the VA ICU team had assumed was being delivered into the patient's stomach ever since the "feeding tube" had been placed. A "feeding tube" that we now knew had been initially inserted into the windpipe, and then forced all the way through the lung tissue out into the space around the patient's lungs. Feeding solution that was not sterile and that proved an ideal medium for the growth of bacteria, leading to a life-threatening, blood borne infection known as "sepsis" and, to add insult to injury, completely collapsed the patient's lung.

Mistakes occur all the time in medicine, especially when residents are involved. It is not truly the residents who bear the responsibility of making sure they know what they are doing. After all, that, by definition, would be impossible, at least some of the time. And so if the VA ICU attendings didn't want to stay late to supervise the placement of a simple feeding tube in a critically ill patient, one would have hoped that there was at least enough thoughtfulness in their supervision of the case that would pick up catastrophic mistakes.

It wasn't so incredible that the relatively inexperienced resident had gotten confused in the middle of the night and had not realized that he had placed the tube into the patient's lung. But what was inconceivable to me was that the attendings who had chosen not to supervise this procedure also hadn't picked up the abnormalities on any of the subsequent chest X-rays as the patient progressively became sicker and sicker—or that the VA radiologists who should have been reading and interpreting the films in parallel with the ICU doctors made the same mistakes.

Neither I nor the Thoracic Surgery Service had been asked to help treat this patient, despite a life-threatening accumulation of fluid inside the chest. Normally, our expertise in this area would have been tapped. My resident had only heard about the case because a friend of his, another young surgery resident, had been the one to emergently place the chest tube that eventually drained the infected mess. My resident was surprised that I had not subsequently been consulted. So was I. It also seemed to me a bit strange that there had been none of the usual VA gossip about a mistake of this magnitude. Then I realized that some of the senior VA medical administrative leadership had been rotating as attendings in the ICU during the management of this patient's case. After that, the paucity of gossip did not surprise me, nor did it surprise me that there was no "comprehensive review."

And ironically, this ICU team may have very well utilized a VA checklist throughout this entire fiasco, and every box would have been duly checked. The resident placed the tube. Check. He ordered a chest X-ray to confirm placement. Check. He bothered to read the film. Check. He even adjusted the tube's position in response to his interpretation of the film. Check. After "confirming" and adjusting proper placement, feeds were initiated. Check. The radiologists subsequently also read the film without raising any concerns. Check. As the patient got sicker, additional X-rays were obtained and evaluated. Check. Fluid was identified in the chest, and was believed to be related to a lung infection. Check. Antibiotics were started. Check. The fluid buildup got worse and the patient arrested.

Checkmate.

CHAPTER TWELVE

Too Good To Be True

In 2005, when I first learned about it from Mark Ratcliffe, NSQIP seemed a straightforward success story. It was a little hard to believe that things in a massive program, implemented on an unprecedented scale across the largest healthcare network in the country's history, had turned out so well. Almost miraculously well. I had forgotten one of the most important lessons I had learned from my fifteen years in the medical business: if something seems too good to be true, it almost certainly is.

In 2005, Mark was clearly enthusiastic about our VA's stellar NSQIP performance. But as years passed, and as his admonitions against risky surgeries became more frequent and more vehement, the NSQIP details that Mark confided to me painted a different story:

1) NSQIP standing had become a critical yardstick used to judge the success of each VA hospital, and the success of local VA administrative leaders;

2) NSQIP standing, like other VA "quality improvement" measures, was also used to determine local VA administrators' annual bonuses; and

3) by 2009 the San Francisco VA's NSQIP results had been dropping steadily, and the hospital no longer enjoyed the coveted status of "low outlier."

Apparently, something dramatic and effective was needed beyond simply pleading with surgeons not to operate on risky patients. It was around that time that Diana Nicoll formed the comprehensive review committee to investigate my practice of thoracic surgery at the San Francisco VA, and shortly after that I was warned by Brian Cason that one more surgical death would end my VA career.

What exactly was NSQIP?[21]

By the 1980s the VA had developed an appalling reputation. So Congress passed in 1986 Public Law 99–166 demanding that the VA measure the quality of its care and determine if it had fallen below "prevailing national standards." But there were two problems: no reliable statistical tools were available to measure the "quality of healthcare," and therefore there was no existing quantitative "prevailing standard" against which the VA could measure itself. Congress therefore gave the VA a very specific mandate instead: to measure its own rates of mortality (death) and morbidity (serious complications) within thirty days of all surgeries, and then compare these numbers to "national standards." These numbers measured just one aspect of VA care, but the selection was seen as a reasonable representation of everything else.

This congressional mandate must have seemed extraordinary to VA leadership, and must have sent a clear message: clean up your act, or else. America's involvement in foreign wars was waning; influential people questioned the need for an enormous and ineffective VA. And so VA leaders, possibly sensing their backs to a wall, devised an unprecedented system to collect data on almost every operation performed, first at selected pilot hospitals, then within the entire VA.

But everybody "knew" that vets were sicker than most "normal" patients, and VA mortality and morbidity were bound to be worse than any "national standard" that could be measured. So the VA took the path of building an unprecedented statistical machine to match its unprecedented mountain of postoperative data, one that determined how many deaths should have been expected during the previous year at each VA hospital. That number was compared to actual deaths that did occur, and an "observed-to-expected ratio," or "O:E ratio," told which

---

[21] For a more in-depth discussion of the origins and implications of NSQIP and other VA quality improvement programs that together form the basis of the so-called "VA Transformation" of the 1990s, see the Appendix.

hospitals performed above average and which hospitals performed below. Still, the VA had no way of comparing itself to a "national standard." This problem must have worried top VA administrators until NSQIP leaders made an astonishing discovery: by simply measuring outcomes, surgical morbidity and mortality began to drop *throughout the VA.*

There had been vague efforts to develop an active quality improvement program out of NSQIP. The "best" hospitals were supposed to report to NSQIP what they thought they were doing right, and NSQIP would try to tell the weaker hospitals how to make their results better. But no comprehensive or coherent intervention program ever appeared. Even if it had, it would have explained improvement only at the worst VA centers, but VA outcomes were improving everywhere. Nevertheless, the VA could tell Congress what it wanted to hear: that VA surgical mortality and morbidity had improved dramatically. In fact, within a decade, they had been slashed by nearly 50 percent. No VA or congressional leader dared question that miracle.

In published articles about NSQIP, VA leaders claimed that employees have a natural tendency to perform better when they know they are being watched. But was it plausible that dramatic, spontaneous improvement had taken place in such a complex process as the delivery of surgical care, a process that involved the interplay of many disparate groups of professionals?

Years before the 2014 VA Waiting List Scandal, in which no organized conspiracy was necessary to account for a remarkably widespread method of administrative deception, I had already begun to wonder if there had not been a far more obvious and more plausible explanation for the "national trend" of ever-improving VA surgical statistics: the withholding of surgery from patients who were likely to have a complication or die. Regardless of how much an individual patient might have needed or deserved the operation. Wouldn't people who were already used to checking boxes to document the value of their work—who were already practiced at making their work *look* satisfactory—find exactly such a way of making their performance look better when they were told exactly what was being watched?

Of course, this "gaming" of the system should have shown up as a drop in the surgical risk factors measured by NSQIP itself. But it turned out that four out of the five most important risk factors in NSQIP were assigned subjectively by the VA doctors who were performing the surgeries or administering anesthesia. Again without implicating any national conspiracy, typical VA practitioners, knowing what was being observed, may have judged their patients to be sicker so that their surgical results would look better. Tell VA doctors that they are being watched, and they may not perform better, but they definitely will try to make outcomes look better.

In 2010, I began to wonder why the VA leadership, Congress, and even the academic community of medical experts who had been exposed to the exaltation of NSQIP hadn't been asking much tougher questions. If the VA interpretation of NSQIP was wrong, and if in fact surgical statistics had been improved primarily by denying surgical care to those who needed it the most, or worse yet by intentionally or even unintentionally manipulating data, then not only was there a crime against scientific integrity, NSQIP was yet another example of the type of abuse of America's veterans that the VA had been asked to answer for in the first place.

> The [Inspector General (IG)] noted that its review of the VHA [in response to the VA Waiting List Scandal of 2014] is ongoing and not confined to Phoenix. The IG is currently investigating at least 42 other VA medical facilities, confirming that "inappropriate scheduling practices are systemic throughout the VHA" and finding "multiple types of schemes used to reduce wait timing data." Furthermore, this is not a recent problem. In 2008, among another dozen reports since 2005, the IG "reported that the problems and the causes associated with scheduling, wait times, and wait lists, are systemic throughout VHA."
>
> –Coburn Report [22]

---

[22] p. 13.

In a June 19, 2013 e-mail directing the staff on how to hide the true wait times of veterans, the Telehealth Coordinator [at the Cheyenne, Wyoming VA Medical Center] told employees who had documented wait lists that they "can still fix this and get off the bad boys list, by cancelling the visit (by clinic) and then re-scheduling it with a desired date within the 14 day window." He explained how every appointment should be recorded to appear to always meet the 14 day goal, even if it did not. "Yes, it is gaming the system a bit," he wrote, "but you know the rules of the game you are playing, and when we exceed a 14 day measure, the front office gets very upset, which doesn't help us."

–Coburn Report [23]

NSQIP was probably viewed as having played a role in saving the VA, if not just the careers of top VA administrators. It may therefore be no surprise that NSQIP results became one of the most important measures against which individual VA hospitals were judged. But the law that created NSQIP, Public Law 99–166, had the far from intended consequence of engendering within the VA an even farther-reaching, powerful defense against any ongoing need for real change in the dismal VA status quo: improvement in "quality of care" statistics. In fact, it wasn't long before a litany of statistics hailed the VA as the best healthcare system in the United States!

In 2009 and 2010, as I was paying increasing attention to reports of the VA's superlative quality of care, I was struck by one of the most remarkable of all VA statistics: the VA outperformed every medical system in the United States on patient satisfaction. At first I could only imagine the poor veterans who populated SF VA waiting rooms every day for hours on end. Then it struck me: the source of the VA's incredible patient satisfaction data was the veterans themselves. The vets are,

---

[23] p. 21.

in general, truly grateful for everything the VA provides. If they had suspicions that patients were treated better or enjoyed better conditions at other healthcare venues, so what? Those people had to pay for that fancy healthcare; the VA was providing services that many vets could not otherwise afford. The vets were not ungrateful, and they'd report greater appreciation for what they got than private patients with much higher expectations, who often and insistently complain about long waits or difficulties getting appointments.

But what about the overall "quality of care"?

In 1995, around the same time the miracle of NSQIP first appeared, the VA also claimed to initiate a "transformation" beyond just improvement in surgical outcomes. Within two years of initiating this "transformation," dramatic improvements were again documented statistically, this time in nonsurgical areas of performance. Again, no mechanism was described that truly explained how the improvement came about. All the VA had begun in 1995 was to measure itself, and to let everyone in the system know exactly what was being measured. In fact, in a paper published in *The New England Journal of Medicine* of May 29, 2003, VA leaders wrote:

> " . . . a systematic approach to the <u>measurement</u> of, <u>management</u> of, and <u>accountability</u> for quality, was at the heart of the improvement. Routine performance <u>measurements</u> for high-priority conditions such as diabetes and coronary artery disease, emphasizing health maintenance and management of care, were instituted. *Performance contracts held managers accountable for meeting improvement goals.*" (Italics added for emphasis.)

In other words, the VA transformation hadn't involved any direct changes in the delivery of care. Instead:

1) changes had been made in the administrative structure of the VA leadership;

2) specific elements of the management of very specific disease processes were carefully measured; and

3) VA administrators were put on notice that the numbers had to improve.

Sound familiar?

Eventually, third-party organizations weighed in with "objective measurements" of the quality of care at the VA and elsewhere; but regardless of who did the measuring, everyone in the VA always knew exactly the few elements that were being observed and recorded.

By 2009, my team and I had long been receiving a tsunami of emails regarding six a.m. blood sugar measurement on the morning after a bypass operation. Why blood sugar measurement instead of the multitude of other post-surgery issues? There was no flurry of emails concerning how much intravenous adrenaline was being infused to keep patients' hearts pumping, or how quickly a neurology consult came to see a patient showing signs of a postoperative stroke. Why blood sugar? And why six a.m.? Six a.m. blood sugars on the day after a bypass, it turned out, were among a limited list of measurements of a limited number of conditions that were collected to assess the overall delivery of inpatient care. Since it was impossible to collect massive sets of data for all of medicine—the way NSQIP had collected massive data just for the two elements of surgical mortality and morbidity—clinical scientists had to assume that measuring specific tiny elements of healthcare delivery would reflect on the delivery of care over a whole system. The problem: the VA always knew exactly which elements were being watched. Did their ability to make these elements look spectacularly impressive mean that a decades-long tradition of mediocre healthcare delivery by a disaffected staff and an immense, indifferent bureaucracy had actually been transformed overnight?

Or had a new VA "tradition" emerged that focused immense energy and attention on the collection of statistics that could be used to deceive Congress and the American people into thinking that everything was fine at the VA, a new tradition that therefore had the effect of actually obviating any need for meaningful change?

According to Brian Turner [a scheduling clerk at a VA health clinic in Texas] . . . good numbers mean better pay and bonuses for employees, especially for upper management. "The financial incentive to meet these measures too easily creates a perverse administrative incentive to find and exploit loopholes in the measures that will allow the facility to meet its numbers without actually providing the services or meeting the expectation the measure dictates. The upshot of these all too widespread practices is that meeting a performance target, rather than meeting the needs of the veteran, becomes the overriding priority in providing care."

–Coburn Report [24]

One day, I heard from a colleague about a complication that the VA's "high quality of care" had not prevented. One of his patients had been doing okay in the ICU, but his blood sugars were persistently elevated. This was not a bypass patient, so dedicated "quality management" personnel were not micromanaging his blood sugar. The ICU doctors had decided to implement a continuous infusion of insulin, an "insulin drip," that could be dialed up or down in response to frequent measurements of the patient's blood.

One night, his nurse decided to make up a new drip. He accidentally grabbed a vial of one hundred units of insulin per milliliter instead of the usual ten. When the patient started on the new drip, he received twenty units of insulin per hour instead of the intended two. Unfortunately for the patient, he had been quite stable for some time on his two units per hour, and he had just had his blood glucose checked before the nurse had changed the drip. The nurse decided that he didn't really need to measure another blood sugar level for several hours, and

---

[24] p. 22–3.

when he finally did so, the blood glucose level, normally between eighty and one hundred thirty, was sixteen.

I had never heard of a blood glucose level that low. I wasn't even sure if that level was compatible with human life. Blood sugar is so crucial to life, and to brain function in particular, that the body has numerous mechanisms to prevent blood sugar levels from dropping that low. Hypoglycemia, the medical term for low blood sugar, is usually quickly reversible, as are its side effects. Usually, there are no lasting complications from a transient drop. But in the history of modern medicine, reports of blood glucose levels below twenty have been infrequent. In fact, massive insulin overdose is one of the few reasons it can happen at all. When blood sugars have been that low for a significant period of time, brain death often results. My colleague's patient, I was told, was in a coma, and people were not optimistic that he would come around.

A nurse at the Lexington [Kentucky] medical center was charged with killing a World War II veteran and eventually admitted fault with very little consequence. The veteran, who served in Europe, was killed by a morphine overdose at a VA Hospital in Lexington, Kentucky in September 2006. The nurse who administered the lethal dose was charged with murder. . . . The court found the "additional doses of morphine provided by" the nurse "were a contributory cause of" the veteran's death and she eventually pled guilty to involuntary manslaughter. At least two other veterans cared for by the same nurse "died under suspicious circumstances" after being given morphine, according to a special agent with the VA Inspector General (IG). The nurse was sentenced to "time served of eight days."

–Coburn Report [25]

---

[25] p. 10.

CHAPTER THIRTEEN

Numbers Can Kill

In April 2010, I returned from family leave and began operating again at the VA. It was a different place from the one I had left. The place had not changed; I had. Not because I had been targeted by the comprehensive review committee. I had a thick skin, and had emerged with my professional standing intact. But for the first time I had become a willing participant in the VA game, and was denying surgery in high-risk cases.

It felt like I had sold out. For an entire year I attended the same clinical conferences that had previously been venues for my crusade to bring cutting edge, aggressive lung cancer care to the veteran's hospital in San Francisco. But now I had become the spoiler.

"I just can't do it," I would tell the oncologists and the pulmonologists who brought their desperate cases to me, hoping to find someone willing to take a chance on their patients' survival.

"They've put our program under a microscope," I would plead, asking my own forgiveness as much as that of any other doctor in the radiology conference room, "and they've told me in no uncertain terms: high risk patients will no longer be brought into the operating room. Period."

From April 2010 until March 2011, none of my patients died, or even suffered a glitch in their postoperative recoveries. I took no pride in this "accomplishment"; instead, for the first time I felt complicit in the veterans' betrayal.

What I thought was a subsequently perfect surgical record, however, proved not to be enough. Ironically, trouble first came from an unexpected direction. Part of the upshot from the "comprehensive review" of my practice at the San Francisco VA was an insistence that greater resources be made available to thoracic surgery, and that I be given some relief for the 100 percent responsibility and the 24/7/365 on-call assignment that I had borne for nearly all of seven consecutive years. One of my colleagues in thoracic surgery at UCSF had already outright refused to continue to come over to the VA. But another colleague agreed to step in and took over about one-third of the operating responsibilities for the service.

Although I didn't lose any of my own patients during the year after my initial inquisition, my colleague did lose two of his patients, both within the span of just one month in February 2011. To be sure, these were difficult and unusual cases—in fact, they were ones that I knew I would have refused to take to surgery myself. Nevertheless, the deaths were enough to feed a new interest in "review"; this time not of my personal practice, of course, but of "thoracic surgery" at our hospital as a whole.

Just at that juncture, in March 2011, it was discovered that one of my senior CT residents, another talented, fully trained general surgeon, had six months earlier closed a two-inch incision on one of my patients, unaware that a two-inch plastic surgical device remained hidden in the tissue below. The veteran had been cured of two separate lung cancers over the course of about one year, both through minimally invasive surgeries that the patient himself described as "painless." But although the patient had not yet suffered negative consequences, a "retained foreign body" was always a very serious surgical complication. Since surgeons generally have no way of knowing when one of the dozens of small needles, sponges, or devices introduced during an operation might lie concealed deep behind tissues in a wound, retention of foreign bodies is normally prevented by means of rigorous counts by OR nurses of every object that goes into the patient, and again when each comes out. A root cause analysis of the event revealed that the foreign body had been retained because of a curious practice among the VA OR nurses: they did not count *disposable* plastic devices. Michael Baker, the nurse responsible, freely admitted that he had therefore failed to count the device.

Although delegating wound closure to the residents was not only acceptable practice but a standard and important element of residents' training and gradual assumption of responsibility, as the attending surgeon in charge, I accepted full responsibility for the complication. And yet, even though my colleague's surgical deaths and the discovery of the retained foreign body in no way indicated substandard practice, all thoracic surgery at the San Francisco VA was put on hold and Diana Nicoll launched another investigation.

* * *

I met William Forrest one afternoon at the San Francisco VA while he was recovering from coronary artery bypass surgery. Though he was fifty-nine at the time, he had a weakened heart and other ailments caused by a tough past life. Like so many of his veteran peers, he looked quite a bit older than his "stated age." He was five feet six or five feet seven and at least fifty pounds overweight. He had obviously been a strong man in his youth; his heavy body was what had remained after chronic heart failure had taken its toll.

Weak heart or no weak heart, William Forrest loved to talk. During the course of several afternoon rounds, I learned that he had grown up in a small town in Missouri, but had hitchhiked his way out to San Francisco just before being drafted into the Vietnam War. He had not been a hippy or a flower child, but he had been fascinated by some of the things he had seen on TV that the young people were doing out in California. It seemed like a different universe from the one in which he had grown up in the rural Midwest. Those young people, he told me, seemed to be thinking for themselves. And even if he thought they were nuts, he admired their courage for letting other people know what was on their minds.

The young Mr. Forrest hadn't gotten to experience much of the Haight-Ashbury scene before his folks let him know, during a long-distance call home, that he had been summoned to report to their local draft board. He ended up becoming an army medic, and was able to use much of what he had learned growing up around farm animals that had constantly gotten into all sorts of trouble. Of course, he doubtless learned a lot more than he had ever wanted to know about pain and suffering while stationed near various Viet Cong strongholds. Nearly forty years later, he still remembered his fascination at realizing that blood was actually water soluble, and that it could be washed out of just about anything with enough soap and elbow grease.

With relatively easy access to all sorts of painkillers during his tours of active duty, Mr. Forrest had been exposed to substance abuse in Southeast Asia that probably made the drug use he observed in psychedelic San Francisco seem like child's play. But he had also been disgusted by some of the wasted life that had gone along with all of that, and after leaving the army, he forced himself back along the straight and narrow path that his parents had attempted to impart to him before their own relatively early deaths.

Whether he had left his heart there just before losing all of his youthful innocence in Vietnam, or whether he just felt he had unfinished business, William Forrest returned not to the Midwest but to San Francisco after coming back from war, and he made the Bay Area his new adopted home. He eventually found work as a mechanic, once again drawing on his experience fixing equipment for his family, his neighbors, and their friends while still in school in Missouri. He married, and at age thirty-two he had a son. While the boy was still in grade school, however, Mr. Forrest and his wife filed for divorce; although often working double shifts to keep up with his child support, Mr. Forrest tried hard to make time every week to shoot some baskets, go hiking, or watch a baseball game with his son.

Mr. Forrest suffered his first heart attack at age forty-eight. He had been working in a small auto repair shop in Rosemont, California, just east of Sacramento, so that he could stay closer to his teenage son. He had been underneath an old VW beetle when the coronary attack hit, and he said he remembered thinking for a moment that the jacks had given way and that the car had landed on his chest. Without realizing it, he had been having bouts of angina for years, as the cholesterol-laden plaques built up relentlessly inside his coronary arteries, occasionally splintering shards of calcified debris into the rushing flow of blood intended to deliver oxygen to his heart. But the chest tightening and mild shortness of breath that he had ignored for years had apparently been nothing compared to the terrifying, crushing pain of true myocardial infarction, and to the overwhelming sense of panic as he felt life itself begin to ebb away from his very grasp.

As soon as he could once again speak from underneath the VW, Mr. Forrest had asked one of his colleagues to bring him to the emergency room at a nearby VA hospital, where the diagnosis of an acute heart attack was made. He didn't remember much of the frightening episode, but he remembered being transferred to the intensive care unit, then out to a quieter hospital bed before being discharged back home. His ex-wife found out what had happened from the other mechanics at the shop, and she brought their son to visit his father as he lay with oxygen tubing pointed up his nose. Although his son was turning out to be a mean tight end on his school's varsity team, Mr. Forrest told me he would never forget the look of fear in the boy's eyes as he watched his father struggle to sit up and use his bedside urinal. That look stuck with Mr. Forrest, and the man vowed never to let his son see him in a moment of weakness again.

Four years after that first MI, William Forrest suffered a second heart attack. This time, he remembered being referred upon discharge from the hospital for cardiac catheterization. After numerous scheduling delays, the catheterization was carried out several months later, and the injection of contrast medium into his small coronary arteries apparently revealed a critical blockage in the vessel that coursed around the right side of his heart. A tiny tubular metal mesh, called a "coronary stent," was placed to open up the severely blocked artery. Mr. Forrest became curious why a cardiac catheterization and stent placement had not been carried out four years before, when this opening up of his artery might have actually prevented his second MI. In response to his queries, he was told by his VA practitioners at that time that at age forty-eight, he would have been "too young" for such a procedure. He was somewhat baffled by the response. If he was old enough to have the disease, he wondered, why would he not be old enough for the treatment? I was unable to shed any more light on what he might have been told and what he might have heard.

Despite his eroding confidence in his VA caregivers, Mr. Forrest had few healthcare choices, and he continued to seek treatment for his progressive heart disease at various VA facilities scattered around the San Francisco and Northern California systems. His worsening angina and his increasing shortness of breath did lead to at least two additional studies over the years, but none of them had resulted in any treatment changes he could remember, and he felt his strength and his stamina wane as his heart muscle was gradually lost to an inadequate flow of blood through his diseased coronary arteries.

$$* \ * \ *$$

Soon after we were barred from scheduling further thoracic surgery at the VA in March 2011, I learned that the 2009 "comprehensive review committee" had not been set up according to the hospital's formal rules, but had been an improvised body pieced together to search for fault among my cases. In 2011, Diana Nicoll did not risk an ad-hoc review process with outside committee members who could escape her control. In accordance with hospital bylaws, Mark Ratcliffe, in his role as the Surgical Service chief, made a formal request to investigate the thoracic surgery section. To achieve that goal, Nicoll formed a review panel, also following hospital bylaw procedure. I learned much later that Ratcliffe's appointment as chair of the three-person review panel, and therefore as chief investigator of his own formal charges, was a violation of legally mandated due process. At the time, I had a lot to learn.

Although it was finally becoming clear to me that I was doing something that the hospital administration did not particularly like, still I found it hard to be too concerned about yet another "investigation." My approach to the previous comprehensive review had been fairly cavalier. I had been confident that my management of difficult cases at the VA had met with a very high standard of care in my specialty, despite the fact that there had been vets whom we weren't able to save. My simple response to that previous inquest had therefore relied entirely on a recital of the truth. That entire affair, in fact, seemed at the time to have been motivated more by an appeasement of an anesthesiologist who in turn may have been driven by his own sense of guilt for endangering a patient. The success of the almost effortless rebuttal I had provided to the insinuation that my care had fallen below some "high VA standard," or that I had exhibited unprofessional behavior, now made it even harder for me to get riled up about these new, even less substantial insinuations.

My naïveté was short-lived. The illusion of objectivity was shattered one afternoon by none other than my "timekeeper," Terry Kerry-Gourneau, who also happened to be Mark Ratcliffe's administrative assistant. She let me know that another surgeon had mentioned to her that a key surgical administrator had asked if he could provide "any dirt on Mann." Assuming that this particular surgeon was not the only one who had been tapped for "dirt," Terry wanted to let me know that some unconventional methods might be at play in the review panel's investigation.

Though I was now clearly the target Nicoll and Ratcliffe were aiming for, actually hitting me presented problems. Since the recent deaths had not been mine, and since the complication in my case was not linked to a deficiency in my practice, the only way they could justify the investigation was to indict the entire General Thoracic Surgery Section, and then hold me responsible as its chief. But that presented yet another problem: there had never been a formal General Thoracic Surgery Section at the San Francisco VA. Thoracic surgery had always been part of the Cardiothoracic Section, and Mark Ratcliffe had always been its chief.

A solution instantly appeared: as soon as the review panel was formed, San Francisco VA paperwork was adjusted, a separate General Thoracic Section leapt into existence, and I was soon receiving formal memos and notifications as its chief. After nearly eight years of trying to advance my too-neglected specialty at the San Francisco VA, I was finally, for the first time, invited to a meeting of the hospital's surgical section chiefs.

Ironically, it was there that I was granted a glimpse of plausible reasons for why the hospital's administration had targeted me and my specialty for elimination. Among the issues reviewed at the meeting were local and national NSQIP data, data that I had never before been given access to. Though I was already aware that our hospital had no longer achieved the coveted NSQIP "low-outlier" status that Mark Ratcliffe had proudly bragged about in years past, I was surprised to see that we had dropped into the third quartile of national O:E ratios—in other words, into the bottom half of one of the most important VA yardsticks of hospital performance. Diana Nicoll must have been profoundly dismayed.

Even more significant to me, however, were the mortality statistics among different surgical specialties throughout the national VA system. The overall mortality average for all types of surgery was about 1.3 percent. As I expected, cardiac and vascular surgery, where patients are often at risk for heart attacks and other life-threatening complications, had higher average mortalities of about 2.15 percent. But by far the single highest mortality, at 3.6 percent, was among thoracic patients, nearly three times the overall surgical average and more than ten times higher than averages for the surgical specialties with the lowest mortalities.

What did that all mean? At around twenty or fewer total deaths in a given year at a hospital our size, the several deaths that could be expected from a busy thoracic service could easily make a significant difference in the hospital's ranking. Many hospitals did not have dedicated thoracic surgeons, which meant that these riskiest of all cases were being concentrated in the ones that did. Furthermore, the risk adjustment model that was generated by NSQIP was based on averages across all specialties, and therefore did not necessarily reflect the peculiar issues among thoracic patients who made up only a small percentage of the total number of patients undergoing surgery in the VA system, but a much higher percentage of the deaths.

Put most simply, if a hospital wanted to reduce its overall mortality, eliminating thoracic surgery yielded by far the biggest bang for the buck. At San Francisco, in order to reduce deaths by the same absolute number, they would have had to eliminate enormous services, such as general surgery or neurosurgery (the latter, of course, was not going to happen at an institution famed for its care of traumatic spinal cord injuries). Cardiac surgery was considered a jewel in any individual VA hospital's crown, and too many vets suffered from severe vascular disease. But lung cancer had always been the black sheep of diseases, the neglected killer. Lung cancer patients in the United States had for many years been underserved and underfunded, often being blamed for bringing on their own catastrophic illness (among VA patients, of course, tobacco use, as a response to the stress of military service, had actually been supported by the military in the form of cigarette rations). It remained true that the vast majority of lung cancer patients throughout the United States, even outside the VA system, were not treated by specialized thoracic surgeons; it would therefore be easy for the San Francisco VA to sneak by without a thoracic specialist. A specialist who would otherwise draw more than the hospital's share of high-risk cases that, statistically, would inevitably drag down its NSQIP results.

If the San Francisco VA had stayed at the top of the NSQIP heap, where it had been before a busy, aggressive thoracic practice was introduced with my recruitment, the hospital's chief of staff and surgical service chief might not have felt pressured to eliminate this riskiest of all surgical specialties from its operating schedule. As the hospital's all-important NSQIP ranking continued to decline relentlessly, however, and as administrative desperation set in, holding on to any sort of thoracic practice must have seemed like a luxury those administrators simply could not afford.

But it wasn't just my continued presence that created a problem. Because all part-time physicians at the VA are given temporary employee status, the San Francisco VA could have fired me at any time without cause. But unusually close ties to UCSF would have left Nancy Ascher and David Jablons feeling obligated to replace me, likely with another young, ambitious candidate bent on continuing an aggressive thoracic practice. The San Francisco VA would be right back where it started.

There was another choice. An investigation into thoracic surgery would put the program on hold. The more drawn out and ugly the process, the longer that hold would last. The beauty of even a "temporary" hold was that doctors would develop other channels for referring thoracic patients to other places. Doctors are creatures of habit, and once established, those new referral patterns would be likely to stick, even after a "temporary" hold was lifted. Even better, a truly ugly procedure, one that not only disrupted a career but that destroyed it, would give both UCSF and potential candidates for my replacement serious pause. And after a "bad experience," San Francisco VA administrators would have much more leverage to say "no" to a candidate they didn't like.

By April 29, 2011, the review panel had already composed its report, a copy of which was, this time, delivered to me promptly. In sharp contrast to the document written by the 2009 comprehensive review committee, which had included only mildly deprecatory innuendo but was for the most part respectful, the review panel report of 2011 was filled with absurd, untrue, and irrational calumny, if not malicious vitriol and libel. Most remarkably, the author of the report seemed indifferent to whether or not there was even the appearance of a rational, objective line of thought. Its seven conclusions stated:

1) *That thoracic mortality at the SF VA was "unacceptably high."* Not true. The data from the report itself documented that there was no statistical difference between San Francisco VA thoracic mortality and thoracic mortality in the rest of the VA system. Even though difficult and risky thoracic cases tended to accumulate at our center, and our mortality should therefore have been higher, it wasn't.

2) *That "sentinel events," as they are called, that occurred during my practice at the VA suggested "a lack of focus and attention to detail."* Not true. Sentinel events in medicine (such as retention of the device that was left inside one of my patients) generally indicate system failures, not individual malpractice. Besides, it was not necessary to ask if sentinel events in my patients' cases "suggested" a lack of focus; after careful analysis by appropriate hospital bodies, they had all been traced to systems problems that were corrected by policy changes. Although they did involve my patients, two of the events had occurred when I had justifiably been away from the patient, making it impossible for a "lack of focus" on my part to have contributed at all.

3) *That my postoperative heart and lung complication rates were higher than those of my colleagues.* Not true. Data in the report itself documented that the rates of these complications were statistically identical. In a bizarre gesture of veiled deference toward the obvious truth, this particular conclusion went on to point out that the demonstration of my higher complication rates might not have been statistically "robust."

4) *That, based on testimony from Michael Baker and my resident, in 2010 I "likely" violated my proctoring agreement* by leaving the operating room while the resident was closing the wound that concealed the retained foreign body. In fact, because enormous attention was paid to the proctoring agreement at the time, if

I had violated it, there would have been an enormous uproar. And in fact, it was standard practice throughout the cardiothoracic specialty for attendings to leave advanced CT residents to close wounds as our cases were winding down. Even if I had left the room at that point, it could not possibly be interpreted as "inappropriate" or "substandard" patient care. Even more to the point, after every operation I had ever conducted, I followed strict hygiene protocol, stepped out of the OR, and washed my hands at the scrub sinks just outside the operating room after removing my surgical gloves. On this case, in accordance with my proctoring agreement, I had immediately returned into the OR with clean hands.

5) *That I was "inconsistent" in managing my time and attendance, indicating a lack of attention to detail in a "critical" administrative area.* Not true. By 2006, Congress and the VA Handbook had both decreed that it was unreasonable for academic, part-time physicians like me to punch a tour of duty time clock. I had specifically been placed on an "Adjustable Work Hours" program that specifically freed me from an unrealistic fixed weekly schedule. In fact, each year I had conscientiously logged my actual hours into the electronic VA system, and each year I was asked to delete hours from my record because I had worked *too many hours* at the VA.

6) *That my management of the thoracic service was "problematic," and that there was "evidence of poor communication between attendings and residents," and that "typically, the attendings do not round on inpatients with residents."* Not true. The report did not provide a single corroborating example of poor communication, and records showed that patient rounds with residents had been performed every day.

7) *Finally, it accused me of the most grievous VA sin: lack of "insight"—* explicitly stating that I opposed the suspension of thoracic surgery at the San Francisco VA (on the grounds that it was an overreaction) and refused to accept responsibility for bad

outcomes. Not true. I had submitted to the review panel in writing my acceptance of responsibility for every negative thoracic outcome that occurred during my VA tenure. And contrary to the generalizations of the report's "conclusions," the review panel's own statistics demonstrated that there had *not* been excess mortality or morbidity on the thoracic service, there had been *no* suggestion of substandard care involved in "sentinel events," and *no* evidence that the management of the service had been in any way deficient. On the other hand, suspending thoracic surgery had an enormously disruptive impact on the care of veterans with life-threatening diseases. Suspending our service had not only been an overreaction, *it was unethical.*

Perhaps the most glaring deficiency in the report was the absence of a single instance of corroboratory evidence or objective documentation for any of the alleged deficiencies. The report had presumably been based on interviews with nine individuals and a review of available data, and yet the accusations were completely undocumented by even a single specific example. Based on its "conclusions," the review panel officially recommended that I be told that my "services [were] no longer needed," and that the one other UCSF thoracic surgeon who was still willing to come out to the VA be put in charge of thoracic surgery in my place.

> In April 2013, [Dr. Jeff] Hawker started work at the Salem Veterans Affairs Medical Center. The center and its five satellite clinics serve more than 110,000 veterans in a 26-county area of southwestern Virginia. . . . The trouble started almost immediately, Hawker said. When co-workers noticed he was putting in long hours, Hawker said they told him several times that he was upsetting contract doctors paid to pick up hours not covered by the staff. Hawker didn't heed the warnings. . . . Soon after [Hawker began lodging concerns with colleagues and superiors about unsafe practices

at the hospital], he got a letter announcing that the hospital would be reducing his salary due to "deficiencies" in his abilities. That letter came just two months after a contradictory letter granting his medical "privileges" after he successfully completed the customary trial period. . . . Things soon worsened for Hawker. He was told his work was being reviewed and he was brought in front of a Medical Executive Board that included some of the people he had mentioned in his concerns. They determined he had made errors in patient care and that he was not qualified for his job. Before the hospital moved to fire him, he was shown a proficiency report signed by [his service chief Rathnakara] Sherigar that gave him an "unsatisfactory" rating for his work during the same time period as Sherigar's earlier review that found him competent to perform his duties. Hawker said he had never been shown the proficiency report until Oct. 17, 2013, three months after the end of the review period listed on the initial report. He suspects the reports were made retroactively to boost the board's case to fire him. . . . The negative review has put "the scarlet letter on my chest," said Hawker, 47.

—Stars and Stripes [26]

* * *

Finally, at age fifty-nine, after years of struggling with the VA for what he felt was a more rational plan to deal with his nagging heart disease,

26 Heath Druzin, "Doctor Says 'Sham Peer Review' Used to Destroy His Career After Pointing Out VA Problems," Stars and Stripes, December 15, 2014, accessed January 25, 2015, http://www.stripes.com/news/veterans/doctor-says-sham-peer-review-used-to-destroy-his-career-after-pointing-out-va-problems-1.319484.

William Forrest ended up at an emergency room at a non-VA community hospital complaining once again of crushing chest pain. This time, however, lab tests ruled out that he was having yet another acute heart attack. That was the good news. But his dramatic change in symptoms was very real, and must have been a reflection of some important disruption of a tenuous equilibrium that had, up until that moment, balanced his heart's need for oxygen and his coronary arteries' ability to provide it.

The doctors in that emergency department were concerned that Mr. Forrest was on the verge of a potentially catastrophic injury to his heart. The administrators of that emergency department became concerned when they learned that Mr. Forrest's only healthcare coverage was through the VA. These administrators were no doubt sympathetic to the urgent needs of our country's veterans, but they also had a fiscal responsibility to their institution. They had almost certainly had numerous unpleasant battles with the VA over both delayed and inadequate reimbursements, or even reimbursements that simply were not forthcoming. Emergency room transfer is a very touchy subject in American medicine, one about which there is an abundance of state and federal law that insists upon the prompt delivery of truly urgent care. But there are loopholes for an emergency room to get potential financial burdens off a hospital's premises and into another hospital's lap; those loopholes generally involve "stabilizing" a patient and then getting the patient's consent to be moved.

One thing was certain from Mr. Forrest's acute decompensation: he was going to need much more aggressive evaluation than the simple "rule out" of an acute MI. He would very likely need invasive—and expensive—tests. The doctor who had been assigned his case laid it on the line and let Mr. Forrest know that if he allowed them to send him over to the San Francisco VA, he would be able to get a comprehensive evaluation and course of treatment in an environment that already understood his situation, and that would follow up diligently on all his future needs.

And so, with Mr. Forrest's hesitant acquiescence, wheels were set into motion, and before too much more time had gone by, he found himself lying in a bed in our state-of-the-art ICU.

The cardiologists at the San Francisco VA certainly did share the outside doctor's concerns about a likely decline in the blood supply to

Mr. Forrest's heart. He was brought soon after his transfer to the cardiac catheterization laboratory, where he was found, to no one's great surprise, to have severe "triple-vessel disease," a condition involving all of the major coronary arteries, and an indication for bypass surgery. He was kept in the hospital on intravenous medications designed to reduce the risk that any of those clogged-up coronaries would shut down completely, and he was brought to the OR fairly expeditiously by one of my colleagues for the bypass from which he might have benefitted even more many years before.

Although, at age fifty-nine, Mr. Forrest finally ended up with several excellent coronary grafts, the years of gradually diminishing blood flow had insidiously and relentlessly weakened the heart muscle upon which the rest of his body depended. At this point, we could tell from ultrasound-based echocardiograms and nuclear medicine studies that large portions of his heart muscle had already died and had been replaced by scar. Other portions, however, were weakened, but might be revived by the sudden increase in blood supply that had been made possible by his grafts. We could tell that these areas in question had not bounced back immediately, but there was still hope. That was the real great promise of the operation—that and the prevention of an unpredictable catastrophic event. But the heart would need time to recover, especially having been set back even further by the abuse and trauma of being operated upon.

Gradually, Mr. Forrest was weaned off of the powerful medications that had kept him alive coming out of the operating room, and, a little more slowly than most, he was eventually ready for transfer out of the ICU. He was able to get by on just a little extra oxygen, but was winded easily just walking across his ward room on his way to the toilet. The pain from his divided breastbone was also harder for him to bear, since fairly chronic medication for lower back pain had made him somewhat resistant to the effects of the painkillers he was being given to help manage the incision down his chest.

As I rounded one afternoon during Mr. Forrest's prolonged stay on our wards, I asked the team if anyone had been coming to visit the middle-aged veteran.

"Well, he's not from around here originally, so he doesn't have much family in this area," the resident began to explain. "He has a niece who lives somewhere in the East Bay, and she's been around to see him once or twice. She travels a lot, though, so most of the time he's all alone."

Just about any patient does better when cradled in the support of those they love. It seemed to me that Mr. Forrest, a garrulous man who obviously thrived on social interaction, would have had a particularly strong need for that kind of caring and psychic stimulation. How, unfortunate, then, and how much harder would it make his recovery, that he was languishing by himself day in and day out in his barren room at the San Francisco VA.

"Wait a minute." I suddenly realized something. "What about that son of his that he likes to talk about? He should be an adult by now. After all that baseball and soccer, you'd think the kid would at least give the man a little of his time."

"Yeah." The resident was ahead of me. "I asked him about his son. Seems the guy lives out in Texas now, and the thing is: Mr. Forrest didn't even tell him he was having this operation. He didn't want to worry him, and I think it has something to do with that story he tells about his kid getting frightened when he had his first MI."

And so, this patient had once again chosen self-sacrifice during his tough and unforgiving life. Mr. Forrest's biggest problem, however, was not his shortness of breath, his incisional pain, or his lack of moral support—it was, instead, a lack of "service connectedness." Eligibility for certain VA benefits was tied to the degree to which a patient had been disabled by service-related injury. It was clear to me and to our service's social worker that Mr. Forrest was not going to waltz out of the hospital after this event. If his heart was going to derive the full benefit of the operation, we were going to need to give it time. And that meant we needed to minimize his extraneous degree of stress and exertion, and that every element of his care needed to remain spot on. Many of our patients would not go straight home after cardiothoracic surgery at the San Francisco VA, but would instead spend time at a rehabilitation center, or at least at a skilled nursing facility, or SNF (pronounced, "sniff"). The problem was, without service connection, and without other documented medical deficits, Mr. Forrest didn't qualify for VA coverage of a SNF.

As usual in these cases, the social worker looked at other possible solutions, but nothing could be found. Mr. Forrest did not himself have the financial resources to pay out of pocket for this type of expensive, round-the-clock care. His niece offered to have him stay with her, which would have been better than nothing, but it was true that her sales job sent her traveling far and wide, and without prior notice of this medical emergency, she had very important conferences on her calendar that would keep her away during the first several weeks of Mr. Forrest's recuperation.

And when anyone would make mention of his son in Texas, the normally jovial Mr. Forrest would become decidedly belligerent, and he refused to allow anyone to violate his HIPAA rights by even contacting the young man regarding his father's predicament.

Although he lived alone, the strict analysis of Mr. Forrest's medical condition dictated that he be sent home according to VA policy. The team dragged its feet, and on postoperative day number twelve, he was discharged home. Amazingly, I subsequently found out from our nurse coordinator that she was not even able to obtain a taxi voucher for Mr. Forrest from the hospital Transportation Office. And so the man was sent off from the San Francisco VA to ride a combination of a bus and two subways to his own small apartment beyond the bay. The nurse and I could only imagine the way he must have reeled in poorly medicated pain from all the jostling, having had his breast bone so recently sawed in two. Considering how winded he was making the trek to his toilet, we shuddered at how he must have struggled, exhausted and gasping for air, as he made his way up to his second-floor apartment.

CHAPTER FOURTEEN

Deus Ex Machina

In April 2011, Diana Nicoll's new, streamlined thoracic surgery review panel, unlike its predecessor in 2009, was quick to deliver a scathing report. There were in it seven condemning "conclusions." The problem was, they were ill conceived, illogical, or contradicted by the very statistical data the panel included as attachments to the report. Many of the complaints were largely administrative, and there was no attempt to back up the panel's "conclusions" with any documented evidence. The entire report was so sloppily put together that it seemed impossible for it to form the basis of any serious accusations, either against the Thoracic Surgery Section or against me.

What I did not immediately realize was that the sloppy nature of the document merely reflected the fact that its contents didn't really matter; I soon learned that its mere existence was all the hospital needed.

I was invited to address the meeting of the hospital's Professional Standards Board (PSB) where the review panel report was reviewed. Only six of the numerous standing members of the PSB were present, including Nicoll, who chaired the meeting, and Brian Cason. I began my presentation with a brief analysis of the mortality and morbidity statistics included in the report. I was somewhat surprised that even this distilled version of the PSB readily agreed that what they had described as the most potentially damning of the review panel's charges, the "conclusions" about my allegedly increased morbidity and mortality, were factually incorrect. Initially encouraged by an apparent willingness to consider the truth, I pressed on at the meeting to refute the other, more subjective "conclusions," many of which involved administrative matters that could not possibly indict my patient care.

One exchange was particularly telling. It related to "conclusion" number six of the review panel report, which decried administrative deficiencies of the "Thoracic Surgery Section"—a section that hadn't even officially existed. In addition to our failure to comply with administrative requirements that did not apply in the absence of an official thoracic section, this conclusion asserted, "There was evidence of poor communication between attendings, attendings and residents, and attendings and consultants." When I pointed out that no corroborating instances of any such "poor communication" were, in fact, described or documented anywhere in the report, Brian Cason, rather indignantly, picked up his copy of the document.

"No, wait a minute," he insisted. "That was in there." He scanned the document for a few seconds, then continued. "Yes, here it is," he said, going on to quote the very same section of the conclusions to which I had drawn their attention. "It says right here 'There was evidence of poor communication between attendings, attendings and residents, and attendings and consultants.'"

I was flabbergasted. Brian had revealed, and in their silence the other PSB members had apparently affirmed, that the conclusions written in the report were, a priori, regarded as gospel. The PSB didn't need or want to be shown any of the evidence that the review panel may or may not have collected. If the review panel report said something was true, then it must have been true. No wonder my attempts at pointing out the deficiencies (in some instances the likely malicious intent) of the report were falling on deaf ears. Given the blistering indictments of the report, the only thing really under consideration at this meeting was how contrite I would appear to be, and how much "insight" I would reflect on my own failures. Which in turn would determine how much my contrition and insight would mitigate the harshness of their verdict.

My "insight" into the veracity of the alleged deficiencies did not come close to appeasing these six members of the PSB. Not long after I left the room, the group not only voted unanimously to endorse the report, they added language taken directly from the hospital bylaws stating that I had "demonstrated behaviors, activities, and professional conduct considered to be detrimental to patient care, to pose a threat to patient safety, to be lower than the standards of the Medical Staff, and to represent inappropriate behavior." Based on that additional conclusion, the PSB recommended that *my privileges to practice medicine at the hospital be revoked*. Despite the fact that the only report conclusions that even suggested a deficiency in patient care, the accusations of increased mortality and morbidity, were accepted to be groundless—and despite the fact that I refuted the other "conclusions"—the six members of the PSB, under the watchful guidance of Diana Nicoll, unanimously called for revocation of my clinical privileges.

I had little knowledge of hospital disciplinary actions. But I knew that revocation of privileges fell on American doctors like an atomic bomb. It was reported to a powerful body, the National Practitioner Data Bank, and could have a catastrophic impact on a doctor's career.

Then came a surprise: Maria Condon, a strong-minded woman who was the only surgeon among the six PSB members to review my case, must have regretted casting her negative vote. The next morning she sent an email to her five PSB colleagues. "During the deliberations," she wrote, "we were rushed, and I felt a certain pressure to conform to the group's ideas." She went on to say:

"The most compelling reason to revoke his privileges, higher morbidity and mortality, were not supported by the evidence. The other crucial issue[,] lax inpatient rounding[,] also had no objective supportive evidence. I take the responsibility of this very seriously. I am not certain that we have sufficient evidence for such an action."

Encouraged by Condon's email, another member of the PSB who had participated in the meeting, a young cardiologist, also objected for reasons "similar to those outlined by Dr. Condon." Diana Nicoll rushed to convene a second PSB meeting later that day. No new evidence was presented, but she insisted that everyone air their views without feeling "rushed." There was another vote that once again recommended revocation; this time, the vote was five to one.

✷ ✷ ✷

From what I was later told, I could surmise that by the time William Forrest had made it home and up the twenty-odd steps to his second-story apartment, all he wanted to do was to throw himself on his unkempt bed and go to sleep. Of course, in his exhaustion-induced slumber, he likely missed numerous doses of his medications, which had been delivered to him in plastic pharmacy bottles collected together in an oversized plastic bag upon his departure from the San Francisco VA. Each of the dozen or so bottles contained a different drug, and on each was written in tiny writing—writing that would have been indecipherable to Mr. Forrest—the hour and dosage at which each of the pills was to be taken. To make things easier, a carefully organized regimen had been composed by the nurses and social worker organizing his discharge, and had been written out on a large piece of paper that he could read. A piece of paper that, when William Forrest emptied out the plastic bag of medicines, did not seem to have made it home across a bus route and two rides on the subway.

Mr. Forrest must have tried to remember at what times he had been taking each of the medicines in the hospital based on the colors and sizes of the different pills. Basically, it was a hopeless proposition. Several of the medications were essential to his recovery. Some, for instance, would regulate the metabolic requirements and the beating of his heart itself; others would modulate fluid accumulation in his lungs, a consequence of the still inadequate function of his cardiac muscle.

Among the most important, of course, was his pain medication. In fact, having missed several doses by the time he woke up at home on the morning of postoperative day number thirteen, the pain in his chest was no doubt excruciating. It would have been sore and bothersome until he coughed, a reflex action that would cause the raw edges of his breastbone to rub against each other, reverberating around the stainless steel wires that had been used to pull his body back together. The pain from this cough was likely more than he could bear, and it might have been at that moment of coughing after first waking up at home that he remembered the red, heart-shaped pillow that he had been given as a gift by the hospital while still in the ICU. Mr. Forrest had been instructed to hold the pillow tight against his chest every time he coughed, because coughing was actually essential for his lung's healthy recovery, and because the pillow could help prevent the incredibly painful movement of the cut edges of his breastbone with each forceful cough. Look though he might again and again in the various plastic bags that he had dragged behind himself on the subway, the red, heart-shaped pillow was simply nowhere to be found.

Mr. Forrest must have been pretty sure which ones were the pain pills—after all, he had been taking similar pills for his back ailments for some time. But it would have been much harder for him to recall exactly which of the plethora of other pills were the ones that were essential to regulate the function of his heart. He likely decided that it was too much to try to deal with the entire pharmacopeia with which he had been sent home, and so he focused instead on getting the most important ones right. He might have remembered one of the nicer nurses, perhaps one with a memorably sweet smile, who always made sure to mention to him that one pill in particular was "the very important one." That medicine took the form of a large, red, oval, translucent pill, very distinctive compared to the others, and so he might have told himself that that was the pill he would make sure to take several times every day.

Realizing that he had been away from home for some time since this ordeal began, Mr. Forrest must have also observed that there was almost nothing in the apartment that he could safely eat. He would therefore have had to gather his strength that afternoon and embark upon a trip to his local grocery for essential supplies. By the time he made it home, he would have almost certainly have been once again too exhausted to even contemplate cooking any of what he had just purchased, and likely struggled instead simply to open up a can of beans.

As Mr. Forrest allowed himself to collapse down for another night of lethargic somnolence, it would have been nearly impossible for him to distinguish how much of his fatigue had truly been due to his exertion, and how much was due to the fact that the delicate balance of heart, lung, kidney, and liver function that had been achieved in the hospital had depended on the carefully devised pharmacologic regimen that now lay in tatters on the floor of his increasingly disheveled apartment.

The recommendation of the Professional Standards Board that my hospital privileges be revoked went next to the hospital's larger and even more influential Medical Executive Committee. That body alone had the authority to recommend revocation of my privileges to the hospital director. The director, in turn, would make the final decision. Again, an imposing Diana Nicoll would chair the meeting of the MEC at which my case was to be discussed.

Just days before my appearance in front of the PSB, I had identified and engaged an excellent medical labor lawyer from Southern California, named David Balfour. After the PSB had sent its recommendation to the MEC, David convinced me to talk to the resident and to the nurse who had reportedly told the review panel that I had on one occasion left the operating room in violation of my 2010 proctoring agreement. It was a standard practice for attendings to leave the OR at that point at the end of an operation, but I had made sure never to do so during the proctoring period. As irrelevant as the allegation might have been to any true question of professional misconduct, it did seem curious that either individual would make such a false incrimination. It turned out, as I had suspected, that the resident had not been asked by the review panel if I had returned to the room after washing my hands. But Michael Baker's response to my inquiry was even more revealing.

"I was never questioned by any review panel," he told me with a very genuine look of incredulity splayed across his face.

I tried to jar his memory, guessing that they might have referred to themselves or to their investigation using some other terminology.

"No, Dr. Mann, I was never interviewed by Dr. Ratcliffe or any of the others you mentioned. Not about you and not about that case. I'm sure of that."

Michael was then very eager to know exactly what testimony had been attributed to him, and he was outraged to find out that he had been falsely implicated in a potentially serious accusation.

"There's no way you could have left the room during all that proctoring business without all hell being raised at the time," he said upon my reading to him the relevant section of the report. "Everyone was paying such careful attention. That's crazy."

He then offered to write a letter in which he documented that he had never, in fact, participated in the review panel investigation. He immediately ran off to his computer and returned with a signed letter in hand. In it he confirmed that he had never been interviewed by the panel, that he had no recollection of my leaving the OR before the end of the case in question, and that his nursing notes would have indicated such a break with the proctoring protocol if it had actually occurred. And although I had not even brought up the problem with the retained piece of equipment, he also chose to add to his letter that the disposable instrument had been left in the patient primarily because he personally had not had a practice of counting such devices while working at the VA.

If sloppiness and sheer statistical incompetence in the preparation of the review panel report had not been enough to demonstrate a malicious bias, fabrication of key witness testimony should have done the trick. And so this time David Balfour himself composed a detailed response to the PSB's report for delivery to the MEC, and we made plans for him to fly up from San Diego and to be present during my appearance in front of the MEC on June 9, 2011.

All for naught. By the time I entered the much larger conference room that was required to hold nearly the entire roster of the hospital MEC, the group had already met to review the case at hand. Although we had been promised that the committee would be given ample opportunity to read and consider the many searing points in Balfour's letter, in fact no such allowance had been made. As I sat down before the group, I could feel the clinical stares that in years past were experienced more commonly by notable cases paraded in front of old-fashioned medical school psychiatry classes. It was obvious that, once again, I was there not to give my side of the story, but to allow the assembly to witness firsthand how deep my pathologic denial ran, and to judge for themselves whether there was any hope at all for my rehabilitation back into their fold.

Though the PSB itself had already rejected the most serious allegations regarding mortality and morbidity, and despite my insistence that innuendo from the review panel report be considered only in the light of a complete absence of documented instances of substandard care or professional misconduct, I left the MEC with little hope of avoiding a recommendation for revocation. Even before we had been notified of the committee's conclusion and of their official recommendation to the hospital director, David Balfour suggested that he relinquish my representation and that I take the case to, as he described them, "bigger guns." Thoroughly discouraged by the little he had witnessed of the MEC "deliberation," he felt pained at the thought that this railroading was very likely to succeed. Our one hope, he believed, was to enlist the help of a famed and legendary godfather of California medical labor law, a San Francisco attorney named Kurt Melchior.

Melchior, it seemed, was an elder statesman and a pillar of one of San Francisco's most revered firms. According to Balfour, he was a wizened litigator, a "member of the California Trial Lawyer Hall of Fame," who had, on numerous occasions, made labor law history and had swayed notable, even infamous cases. His name alone, as David put it, might send a message to the lawyers who were employed in the local VA legal department, and who had been providing guidance and reassurance to Diana Nicoll. The hope was that his reputation might be enough to instigate a hiccup in Nicoll's otherwise flawless execution of a baseless lynching.

I only hoped that this Kurt Melchior would know what he was doing.

✳ ✳ ✳

After a couple more days of exhaustion, and noticing a progressively rapid deterioration into worse and worse shortness of breath with less and less vigorous exertion, Veteran William Forrest, attempting to recover by himself at home from a coronary bypass operation complicated by chronic heart failure, had decided to seek help from a local VA clinic. There had been a community VA outpost not far from where he lived, where he had gone on several occasions seeking additional pain medication for his back, and where he had, at times, gotten his toenails attended to by a podiatrist who would rotate through.

Mr. Forrest must have taken his time to get to the clinic, riding one bus and stopping frequently to rest during the pedestrian portion of the journey. Upon his arrival, he checked in with the front desk staff and told them that he was concerned because he had just had a bypass operation and didn't feel too well. Attempting both triage and differential diagnosis, the staff personnel would have asked him what was bothering him most, to which he honestly replied the pain down the middle of his chest.

The staff member then likely asked him to take a seat in the waiting area, and after dealing with other matters on her desk, pulled up his file from the clinic records. Discovering that he had been ascribed a pattern of "drug-seeking behavior" in the past, I was later told that she became suspicious of the veteran's claim of postsurgical pain. Uncertain of how to handle the situation, she asked one of the nurse practitioners, who was at the time the practitioner in charge.

"Well, if he's just had a CABG," the nurse replied, "we should at least make sure this chest pain is not from an MI. Let's do an EKG and draw a troponin to rule him out."

The computerized analysis of Mr. Forrest's EKG indicated that the study was "abnormal," but the nurse practitioner was experienced enough to know that EKGs were always abnormal during the post-op recovery from heart surgery. Nothing about the EKG looked like an acute MI to her. It would take a little more time for definitive blood tests to come back from the outside laboratory, but she went to talk to the patient to see if she could let him wait at home for the likely negative results.

"Your chest hurts, doesn't it, Mr. Forrest?" the nurse said in a sympathetic voice.

"Oh, something awful."

"Well, you know, your color looks good and this EKG looks just fine, and it's really very normal for people to have pain in their incisions after a big operation like yours."

And so, after a pat on the back and instructions to keep taking the pain medicine that had been prescribed in the hospital, William Forrest was sent back home, hoping he would get there in time to take that big translucent red pill before he had fallen even further behind his medication schedule.

✳ ✳ ✳

I first met Kurt Melchior and one of his talented younger associates, a former doctor named Gregg Cochran, at the dizzying height of their offices in a skyscraper in downtown San Francisco. The majestic floor-to-ceiling view of San Francisco Bay, Alcatraz Island, the Marin Headlands and, of course, the Golden Gate Bridge, provided an incongruously peaceful and calming backdrop to the nightmarish conversation we were about to have. Four days before that meeting, I had been informed, face-to-face, by Ratcliffe and Nicoll that the MEC had decided to recommend the revocation of my clinical privileges. Now, Kurt Melchior was about to let me know what that really meant.

"Once the state medical boards where you hold your licenses are notified that a hospital has revoked your clinical privileges," Kurt said, realizing that he was addressing someone truly uneducated with regard to matters of medico-legal discipline, "the boards will look into the matter, but they almost never take opposition to the hospital's action." His gruff voice reinforced the impression that he'd been around many blocks, and his straightforward manner of speaking suggested that he had gained a formidable amount of wisdom along the way. "In fact," he continued in his matter-of-fact tone of voice, "they will almost always respond by revoking your license to practice medicine."

"You're kidding, right?"

"I wish I were." Kurt Melchior had clearly needed to train himself over the course of a long and trying career to deliver bad news in a sympathetic but effective way. It was all too reminiscent of what I had needed to learn myself.

"But couldn't we ask the Medical Board to take a closer, more rational look at the merits of what had been done?"

"There are avenues to request a review, but they almost never succeed."

Somehow, I had gotten to this point, almost to the end of an excruciating rope, without having discovered this most salient of details. I had heard of "reportable events" at various times during my medical education and academic career, but had never gotten near enough to one that involved either myself or any of my close colleagues. I didn't really know anything about this National Practitioner Data Bank to whom "reports" were made, and I knew even less about what was done with the information. I had realized, however, that there must have been good reasons why they were such dreaded events; I had no idea that they entailed professional annihilation.

On the other hand, the people at the San Francisco VA who were pursuing this course of action, and in particular Diana Nicoll and Mark Ratcliffe, could not possibly have been as oblivious as I to the menacing reality of the revocation's implications. They must have known all along that revocation of privileges would lead directly to the loss of my medical license. And they must also have known that without that license, my continued appointment on the faculty at UCSF would be impossible, as well. My entire career would come to a crashing halt: decades of commitment and hard work, of developing skills to help underserved groups of patients, of building a cutting edge research program, of finding new and better ways to save lives and to minimize suffering—even attempts to spread these types of advances around the globe—would all be lost. And all that was on top of the catastrophic impact on my own family.

Nor were Diana Nicoll or Mark Ratcliffe complete idiots. They had tried diligently to come up with reasonable justifications for this professional assassination, and in the absence of any they had decided to proceed with empty accusations in a series of kangaroo courts. They had tried hard and had failed to find any true indictment of my practice of surgery; that failed undertaking was itself an ironic and powerful corroboration that I must, in fact, have been doing something right. By subjecting me to repeated inquisition and by hearing my repeated defense, they had also learned in detail of the consistent success of my clinical practice in a similarly challenging and high-risk patient population at UCSF. If they truly hoped to find a few good people to help their veterans fight life-threatening disease, wasn't I their man, even if I wasn't the most reverent follower of their "policies"?

And yet here they were, knowingly hell-bent on my professional destruction. Had they simply wanted to stop me from bringing high-risk cases into their OR, they could have asked me to leave. As a part-time VA physician, I would have no choice. We had no employment guarantees, not even any right to appeal employment decisions. But while merely discontinuing my contract and sending me on my way could have brought temporary relief to those who worried most about the San Francisco VA's NSQIP standings, it must not have seemed like a definitive enough solution. It was quite possible that David Jablons, Scot Merrick, and Nancy Ascher would recruit another, even more aggressive young thoracic surgeon in my place. A very visible and "violent" lynching, on the other hand, would send a much clearer message about what Diana Nicoll would and would not tolerate. The protracted administrative spectacle itself put a prolonged hold on having any thoracic surgery performed at the San Francisco VA. Ratcliffe and Nicoll knew very well that that type of hiatus would be long enough for referral patterns to shift and for VA doctors around Northern California to figure out other ways of having their lung cancer patients operated on. Even more importantly, my ugly professional disembowelment would throw frigid water on the eagerness of UC surgeons to recruit a successor, and on the appetite that any other aggressive thoracic surgeon might otherwise have had for this position in San Francisco.

So here we were, thirty stories above the hilly streets of San Francisco, with fresh cups of coffee in our hands, facing an eleventh-hour uphill battle against an almost inexorable, predetermined outcome. That was when the similarities between my practice of thoracic surgery and Gregg and Kurt's practice of the law became most obvious to me. They were willing to use appropriate diagnostic phrases, such as "hopeless," or "bleak," but they showed no willingness at all to give up hope. I had been sent to them, just as so many patients, refused treatment by other surgeons, had been sent to me. Between the two of them, they had more than forty years of experience battling medical labor cases, both defending accused doctors and prosecuting them on various hospitals' behalves. They were no light-hearted dilettantes, nor had there been much they hadn't seen before. Nevertheless, as the two quickly came up to speed on the details of my affair, they just as quickly became personally incensed by what they learned. They told me that for them, my situation had crossed a line. It was no longer simply an interesting case, it had become more of a personal crusade. In one email, Kurt would later write to Gregg and to me, "This absolutely goes beyond the defense of 1 doctor: it deeply offends my sense of fair play."

But at that first meeting, soon after I had been told of the MEC verdict, we had little to go on and had not yet come up with much to put forth. Their first, almost instinctive tactic was to buy time, especially since the written notice I had received from Nicoll on July 11, 2015, provided only ten days for a complete, written response to the hospital director regarding the MEC's recommendation. Buying time proved easy enough—Gregg immediately identified several glaring omissions from Nicoll's letter that were required by the hospital's own bylaws of such an official notification. It should have been a simple thing to correct the "Notice of Intent," and yet it wasn't until August 26, one and a half months later, that the VA legal team had composed a notice that fulfilled all of their own bureaucratic requirements.

What Kurt and Gregg demanded of this letter, and what the VA legal department struggled to provide, was a clear and specific description of what the MEC was accusing me of having done wrong. To Kurt and Gregg, the case was a witch's cauldron of bizarre and absurd elements, the most bizarre being the VA's failure to identify a single instance of substandard behavior or practice on my part. In their experience, such instances had always been the basis for—and the central element of—these types of proceedings. Furthermore, without a clear description of the exact charges, a doctor could not reasonably defend himself in the letter he was allowed, also according to the bylaws, to write to the hospital director.

In the end, the revision of Nicoll's official letter could point only to the "sentinel events," the complications that had occurred during a few of my cases that were found on analysis to have resulted from systemic problems in the *hospital's* delivery of care. Even the VA lawyers must have known that without any evidence that malpractice on my part had contributed to these events, the events themselves could not have presented legally sound grounds for action against me.

The hospital also provided a transcript of the MEC meeting (again according to hospital bylaws). This proved to be another witch's cauldron of absurdities. For starters, Mark Ratcliffe had not only been appointed to lead an investigation of his own charges, but was assigned to provide the MEC with an "objective" review of the investigation's findings. As the accuser, he should never have participated in an impartial MEC deliberation, much less lead it. Even worse, the MEC discussion violated state and federal requirements of due process. From its opening moments, the meeting had avoided objective discussion of actual facts uncovered by the review panel. As Kurt and Gregg wrote to Hospital Director Lawrence Carroll, instead, it was "an entirely subjective and uncorroborated tirade against Dr. Mann by the very individual who had raised the initial accusations and then had been put in charge of investigating his own charges . . . a subjectively horrific and completely unsubstantiated portrayal of Dr. Mann."

∗ ∗ ∗

William Forrest made it home in one piece from his visit to the local VA outpatient facility, but just barely. Over the next day or so, as his heart and his body fluids fell inexorably further and further out of balance, his lungs found it increasingly harder to extract oxygen from the air and to deposit it into his blood. His kidney shutdown was a direct result of the paucity of blood flow that they received from his failing heart, and of the poor oxygen content of the blood that did make it through. Without a pair of functioning kidneys, the fluid buildup in his lungs progressed even faster, and the downward spiral accelerated.

Mr. Forrest continued to decline, and the former soldier inevitably became profoundly short of breath. He might have thought about returning to the VA outpatient clinic, or even about trudging all the way back to the San Francisco VA hospital. With legs that had swollen up to the size of small tree trunks, however, he could no longer have gotten himself out the apartment door, much less across San Francisco Bay.

Luckily, before he began to lose consciousness, he remembered that the discharge instructions he had received included an "800" number that he was instructed to call in case anything went awry after his return home. The hotline was part of an attempt to streamline VA management of postoperative discharges and avoid unwanted "bounce backs." The number had seemed so important to the nurses that he remembered having folded the card on which the number had been printed and placing it directly into his wallet.

William Forrest dug his wallet out of the pocket of his trousers, and sure enough he found the number printed on the folded card. With little else at his disposal, he called the number and held on as the phone on the other end rang. Finally, when the call was answered, a recorded voice had told him that his call was important, and that it would be answered in the order it was received.

Likely dozing off intermittently with the phone on his ear, Mr. Forrest must have waited until a human being finally picked up his call. To the best of his ability, he attempted to explain his situation. He was asked to verify his call back information, was thanked for using the 800 hotline, and was told that someone would call him back.

Another several hours went by, and Mr. Forrest decided to give the number one more try. After a similar delay on hold, his call was once again answered, and this time he immediately began to plead for help. After being calmed down enough to once again provide his last name and the final four digits of his social security number, Mr. Forrest was reassured that they had received all the necessary information, and that a qualified practitioner would soon call him back.

✶ ✶ ✶

Kurt Melchior and Gregg Cochran eventually composed a sixteen-page letter, spelling out to San Francisco VA Hospital Director Lawrence Carroll all the elements of my case. It did not merely request fair consideration of our position; it implored him to stop the VA from proceeding down an illicit path that had already undermined my constitutional rights. Still, we had little hope that Carroll, a businessman, would reject the nearly unanimous recommendation of dozens of his hospital's medical experts who had all signed off on the PSB and MEC "deliberations."

For months my lawyers had delivered powerful arguments on my behalf to the local VA's legal department—and achieved nothing in return. While we waited for a response from Lawrence Carroll, I made good on a promise to Nancy Ascher to keep her informed and sent her a copy of the sixteen-page letter. She was outraged and immediately brought the letter to UCSF's chief counsel, who immediately brought it to the dean of the medical school. Later that day, the dean made a phone call to Carroll, and that afternoon, my lawyers received word from the VA legal department that the proceeding would be completely dropped.

Deus ex machina. Like a god suddenly appearing onstage to resolve impossible predicaments at the end of an ancient Greek play, the dean stepped in from nowhere and ended my six-month ordeal. This sudden turn of events was so improbable it teetered on the edge of impossible. But it saved my career.

It was only later that I learned that other VA doctors had been subjected to disciplinary actions that jeopardized their careers after they resisted or objected to practices at their hospitals. Local VA legal departments are always involved in such actions, and if "sham peer reviews," as they have come to be known, are as widespread as they seem to be, it is hard to imagine that the Central VA legal department is not aware of them, as well. There were easier ways for the San Francisco VA to get rid of me if they didn't like what I was doing; instead, I was caught up in a pattern of VA abuse that was directed not just at veterans, but at people who try to serve those veterans to the fullest.

NSQIP was instigated by a congressional demand for improved veteran care. In stark contrast, the most plausible explanation for the "miracle" of NSQIP nationally was that surgical care was subsequently withheld from veterans whose cases threatened the statistical reengineering of the VA's façade. Locally, Diana Nicoll pushed a recommendation for the revocation of my privileges through a process that violated my constitutional rights, all under the watchful eye of VA lawyers, at a time when the VA hospital she led was critically concerned about the impact of high-risk operations on its all-important NSQIP ranking.

And although I was in a better position to defend the integrity of my career—or perhaps just luckier—than many innocent doctors who have been targeted by the VA, the local San Francisco VA strategy was essentially successful. Once thoracic surgery was put on hold in 2011, it was more than two years before another surgeon was brought on who could handle thoracic cases. To this day there is no general thoracic surgical specialist at the San Francisco VA and no aggressive lung cancer program. Only a handful of the thoracic cases have been performed each year, and no likely change is in sight.

> James Martin, a doctor and national representative for the American Federation of Government Employees, said he is working on multiple cases of sham peer reviews in which VA doctors have been forced out by unethical administrators. "I've got all kinds of stories," he said. According to Martin . . . it's fairly easy for administrators to oust doctors because the entire process is done in house. Doctors who report wrongdoing or malpractice are often judged by the very same people they have criticized. . . . "There's a cloak of secrecy that gives them the power to do these things without transparency," he said about the current in-house process.
>
> *—Stars and Stripes* [27]

---

[27] Heath Druzin, "Doctor Says 'Sham Peer Review' Used to Destroy His Career After Pointing Out VA Problems," Stars and Stripes, December 15, 2014, accessed January 25, 2015, http://www.stripes.com/news/veterans/doctor-says-sham-peer-review-used-to-destroy-his-career-after-pointing-out-va-problems-1.319484.

* * *

Two days after William Forrest's call to the VA 800 post-discharge hotline was duly recorded, a nurse from the hotline finally followed up and called in to Mr. Forrest's apartment. The phone was answered not by the veteran, but by his niece, who had returned during a hiatus in her out-of-town business meetings, and who was in the apartment completing arrangements for her uncle's wake. Upon further questioning, the nurse was informed that the young woman had found the veteran dead in a pool of his own frothy saliva two days before, lying near the phone, grasping a half-empty bottle of stool softeners that had come in the form of oval, red, translucent pills.

> Rushed by his family to a Phoenix, Arizona VA emergency room in September 2013, [a Navy veteran with bladder cancer] was sent home, even though his medical chart said his situation was "urgent." According to reports, the VA never called to schedule a follow-up appointment, so the veteran and his daughter-in-law called "numerous times" to get the urgent appointment for him. She says she called "day after day" for months, but the response was never helpful. "Well, you know, we have other patients that are critical as well," she was told. "It's a seven-month waiting list. And you're gonna have to have patience." After enduring months of agonizing pain and suffering, he died on November 30, 2013. She said the VA finally returned the calls to schedule an appointment on December 6 – one week after her father-in-law had died.
>
> —Coburn Report[28]

---

[28] p. 8.

CHAPTER FIFTEEN

The VA Way—Today

My exposure to VA hospitals in Palo Alto, Boston, and San Francisco, even before I began my tenure as a VA staff surgeon, gave me a strong sense not only of the unique features of each of these prominent, highly regarded VA facilities, but also of features common to the institution as a whole. There were clearly attitudes and experiences that were shared both by patients and practitioners throughout the system. I have related my experiences that best exemplify these system-wide trends, and that particularly reveal the reality of the current day Veterans Health Administration.

The stories in this book, however, are limited to what I witnessed firsthand, primarily at one VA hospital (though one often cited as among the VA's very best). And the VA successfully ended my exposure to its system in the fall of 2011. Throughout the book, I have therefore included excerpts from third-party accounts of other alarming stories that have occurred throughout the VA system, many of which took place after I left the San Francisco VA.

The following quotations provide additional examples, taken largely from Senator Tom Coburn's extensive oversight report from 2014, that corroborate a picture of the VA that remains largely unchanged to this day:

Synopsis

Too many men and women who bravely fought for our freedom are losing their lives, not at the hands of terrorists or enemy combatants, but from friendly fire in the form of medical malpractice and neglect by the Department of Veterans Affairs.[29]

Split-second medical decisions in a war zone or in an emergency room can mean the difference between life and death. Yet at the VA, the urgency of the battlefield is lost in the lethargy of the bureaucracy. Veterans wait months just to see a doctor and the Department has systemically covered up delays and deaths they have caused. For decades, the Department has struggled to deliver timely care to veterans.[30]

Over the past decade, more than 1,000 veterans may have died as a result of VA malfeasance.[31]

The waiting list cover-ups and uneven care are reflective of a much larger culture within the VA, where administrators manipulate both data and employees to give an appearance that all is well.[32]

Good employees inside the VA who try to bring attention to problems or errors are punished, bullied, put on "bad boy" lists, and transferred to other locations. These whistleblowers who come forward to expose the problems demonstrate many employees within the VA are dedicated to serving veterans and willing to put their livelihood at risk to ensure our nation's heroes are getting the care they were promised.[33]

Too many veterans who rely upon the VA are stuck in a bureaucratic maze that is inconvenient, unaccountable, inefficient, and limits choices with varying outcomes.[34]

This has created an environment where veterans are not always the priority. For example, the Department suffers from a shortage of health care providers; yet, the VA pays nurses to perform union duties and allows doctors to leave work early rather than care for patients. It

---

[29] Coburn, p. 4.

[30] Coburn, p. 4.

[31] Coburn, p. 4.

[32] Coburn, p. 4.

[33] Coburn, p. 5.

[34] Coburn, p. 5.

also tolerates employees skipping work for long periods of unapproved absences, while veterans cannot get phone calls answered or returned.[35]

Numbers

Out of the current veteran population of more than 21.6 million, more than 9.1 million veterans are enrolled in the VA system.[36]

With over 288,000 employees, the Department provided medical care to over 6.4 million patients in 2013.[37]

The VHA's central office staff has grown markedly—from about 800 in the late 1990s to nearly 11,000 in 2012.[38]

Substandard VA care

At least 82 vets have died or suffered serious injuries as a result of delayed diagnosis or treatment for colonoscopies or endoscopies at VA facilities. After investigating these deaths, CNN could not determine whether any VA employee has been fired or even reprimanded for these failures. In fact, "some of the people responsible may have even received bonuses in recent years for their work, despite the delays in care or treatment for the veterans."[39]

In total, 5,100 veterans in need of gastrointestinal procedures went without consultations between 2011 and 2012 in Georgia. These included a delay in 2,860 screenings, 1,300 surveillance and 340 diagnostic endoscopies.[40]

Suicides occurred among mentally ill patients as they waited in between appointments that were scheduled long in advance, fraudulently made to look as if they were given within 14 days of a "desired" date.[41]

Mrs. Jerletta Halford-Pandos is a 100% disabled veteran from Kellyville, Oklahoma. Mrs. Halford-Pandos, who served her country

---

[35] Coburn, p. 5.

[36] Coburn, p. 6.

[37] Coburn, p. 6.

[38] Coburn, p. 6.

[39] Coburn, p. 8.

[40] Coburn, p. 9.

[41] Coburn, p. 12

from 1980–2002, had both of her knees replaced by the VA—twice each. On her second knee surgery on her left knee, the VA placed a 5-inch rod in her femur, which extended her leg one inch. The VA failed to notify Mrs. Halford-Pandos that the rod would extend her leg—until six months into her physical therapy. "It would have been nice if they (VA) would have told me," she said.[42]

In 2007, military veteran Christopher Ellison visited a Philadelphia VA facility for a routine tooth extraction. Suffering a stroke on his way home, because doctors performed the procedure despite Ellison's dangerously low blood pressure, he is now permanently paralyzed.[43]

Thaddeus Raysor, an Army veteran, reported to a VA hospital yearly for chest x-rays. For three years, VA staff failed to diagnose a growing lesion in his lung – which ultimately killed him.[44]

At a South Carolina hospital, one veteran had to wait nine months for a colonoscopy, and by the time he had the surgery, he was diagnosed with Stage 3 cancer. The VA admitted this was "a significant delay," and had the procedure been performed earlier, his cancer may not have been so progressive.[45]

Excessive waits for VA care

The VA has a five-day timeliness goal to complete hearing aid repair services, which is typically exceeded by 15 days, and 30 percent of veterans are forced to wait more than a month. At the VA's Denver Acquisition and Logistics Center (DALC), OIG [Office of the Inspector General] investigators found "about 19,500 sealed packages of hearing aids waiting for repair and for staff to record the date received from veterans and medical facilities into the production system. Without timely recording of the date DALC received a hearing aid, repair staff cannot identify if the veteran's hearing aid was received or report on the status of the repair."[46]

---

[42] Coburn, p. 19

[43] Coburn, p. 19.

[44] Coburn, p. 19.

[45] Coburn, p. 19.

[46] Coburn, p. 23.

The VA canceled over 1.5 million medical orders for veterans "without any guarantee the patients received the treatment or tests they needed. You don't know whether people received the care or if they received it in a timely manner. There's no audit trail. There's no way to know whether they were appropriately closed," said GAO's health care director Debra Draper. GAO's review found numerous cases of consults being closed without clinical reviews or services being provided.[47]

"114 VA medical facilities limited access to purchased home care services through the use of more restrictive eligibility criteria than required." In addition, "VA facilities did not use required waiting lists to track eligible veterans." The OIG concluded the problem was a result, in part, of a lack of oversight in program management and "affected the care received by Veterans and sometimes resulted in the denial of care."[48]

The VA's "Corrosive Culture"

The department has a history of retaliating against whistle-blowers, which Sloan D. Gibson, the acting V.A. secretary, acknowledged this month [June 2014] at a news conference in San Antonio. "I understand that we've got a cultural issue there, and we're going to deal with that cultural issue," said Mr. Gibson. . . . The federal Office of Special Counsel, which investigates whistle-blower complaints, is examining 37 claims of retaliation by V.A. employees in 19 states, and recently persuaded the V.A. to drop the disciplining of three staff members who had spoken out. Together with reports to other watchdog agencies and the Times interviews, the accounts by V.A. whistle-blowers cover several dozen hospitals, with complaints dating back seven years or longer.[49]

Dr. Jacqueline Brecht, a former urologist at the Alaska V.A. Healthcare System in Anchorage, said in an interview that she had a heated argument with administrators at a staff meeting in 2008 when she objected to using phantom appointments to make wait times appear shorter, as they had instructed her. She said that the practice amounted to medical fraud, and complained about other patient care problems

---

[47] Coburn, p. 19.

[48] Coburn, p. 23.

[49] Eric Lichtblau, "V.A. Punished Critics on Staff, Doctors Assert," *The New York Times*, June 15, 2014, accessed June 17, 2014, http://www.nytimes.com/2014/06/16/us/va-punished-critics-on-staff-doctors-assert.html.

as well. Days later, a top administrator came to Dr. Brecht's clinic, put her on administrative leave, and had security officers walk her out of the building. Dr. Brecht, who was put on leave, said she thought about calling a whistle-blower's hotline at the time, but feared that administrators might take further steps to discredit her and risk her medical licensing.[50]

At the V.A. Medical Center in Wilmington, Del., Michelle Washington, a psychologist treating soldiers with post-traumatic stress disorder, also found her worries unwelcome. She said in an interview that she faced retaliation when she testified in 2011 to a Senate committee about staffing shortages that she said left veterans waiting dangerously long for psychological help. A week before her scheduled appearance, Dr. Washington said she received an evaluation downgrading her performance at the hospital from "outstanding" to "unsatisfactory," citing management complaints she had never heard before. She was also stripped of some psychological treatment duties. "I'm not sure how I went from outstanding to unsatisfactory in 30 days," Dr. Washington said. "The only intervening thing was my testimony."[51]

"The V.A. isn't a place where you speak out," Dr. [Janet] Stout, [former VA infectious disease specialist] said in an interview.[52]

A VA tradition of obfuscation makes conspiracy to produce misleading statistics unnecessary; it is the natural "VA way"

The initial stages of the audit found "a systemic lack of integrity" throughout the VHA health care system. The final audit confirmed inappropriate scheduling practices across the Department finding that "57,000 veterans have been waiting more than 90 days for an appointment." . . . Two different types of illicit scheduling practices were discovered in at least one instance in 70% of VA facilities, often linked to administrator bonuses. Most concerning, VA had ample opportunity to improve these scheduling deficiencies, but often chose not to do so.[53]

---

[50]   Lichtblau, *The New York Times*, June 15, 2014.

[51]   Lichtblau, *The New York Times*, June 15, 2014.

[52]   Lichtblau, *The New York Times*, June 15, 2014.

[53]   Coburn, p. 14.

A former employee of the Los Angeles VA Center and Marine veteran, Oliver Mitchell, said he "was instructed to help cancel backlogged veteran medical exam requests during a coordinated process that began at the facility in March 2009." Mitchell said, "There was no selective review. There was a list that went back to the '90s and they just went through and canceled each one." The interim service chief at the Los Angeles VA hospital's radiology department told schedulers "she was under pressure from VA headquarters to reduce the backlog." She said "her job was on the line and that this would be the death of her if we didn't delete and/or cancel any of the pending backlog," according to Mitchell.[54]

Nick Tolentino, a retired Mental Health Administrative Officer at the Manchester VA Medical Center in New Hampshire revealed he and others were expected to lie about medical services that were not provided. He said, "We were never to answer that services were not provided. Many of the answers were changed to say that specific (required) services WERE being provided when they weren't. Specifically, we were instructed that the 'fallback' answer was that the services were provided by fee-service, although this was never actually the case." Mr. Tolentino said VA staff would conspire internally and with other VA centers to find loopholes around performance metrics. He noted, "it was a routine matter for facility and VISN administrators to find and use loopholes to 'meet their numbers' whenever they were confronted with a gap between a performance requirement and a facility's limited capabilities that had adverse implications for their paychecks. Tragically, this 'gaming' of the system meant that veterans too often were not receiving necessary health care services." It "was made clear to us in a meeting that the service line priority needed to be 'quantity' rather than 'quality.' By that she meant to 'have contact with as many veterans as we can, even if we aren't able to help them.'"[55]

At a VA medical center in New York City, hospital administrators pressured surgeons to admit patients to keep overall patient numbers high. "The practice became so abusive," wrote one former physician at the facility, "that one day a man arrived on the hospital inpatient floor

---

[54] Coburn, p. 21.

[55] Coburn, p. 22.

carrying admission papers specifying a diagnosis of appendicitis. When my fellow residents and I asked him what was wrong, the patient said he didn't know; he had come for a routine clinic appointment without complaints, and a woman (the attending surgeon) handed him the paperwork and directed him to go upstairs. He denied having abdominal pain and reported having had an appendectomy 15 years earlier."[56]

ASPIRE is one database buried on the VA's website that provides certain metrics for each Veterans Integrated Service Network (VISN). Over half the metrics – mostly those related to timeliness of care and patient satisfaction – are listed as "not yet available" with no indications of when such data will be published. The LinKS database shows how hospitals are doing in a number of process measures, but the criterion used to determine the score essentially always allows facilities to receive a passing score.[57]

A former VA official revealed the perverse financial incentive for VA employees to earn bonuses by cleverly hiding the number of wait listed veterans: "First and foremost, the achievement of performance measures is linked to pay and bonuses for Executive Career Field (ECF) employees, most commonly, upper management (myself included). The financial incentive to meet these measures too easily creates a perverse administrative incentive to find and exploit loopholes in the measures that will allow the facility to meet its numbers without actually providing the services or meeting the expectation the measure dictates. The upshot of these all too widespread practices is that meeting a performance target, rather than meeting the needs of the veteran, becomes the overriding priority in providing care."[58]

---

[56] Coburn, p. 26.

[57] Coburn, p. 25.

[58] Coburn, p. 29.

APPENDIX

NSQIP

When I had first learned about NSQIP from Mark Ratcliffe, it sounded like a straightforward success story. Yes, it was a little hard to believe that things in a massive program, implemented on an unprecedented scale across the largest healthcare network in the country's history, had turned out so well. Almost miraculously well, in fact. But at the time, it was basically yet another VA bureaucratic reality, one that I was inclined to ignore if it did not impact directly upon my already difficult work. I had forgotten one of the most important lessons I had learned from my fifteen years in the medical business: if something seems too good to be true, it almost certainly is.

But if Mark was ebullient over NSQIP in those days, he had good reason to be. He felt it had provided absolute proof of the supremacy of the San Francisco VA's surgical program. After all, San Francisco had been the only hospital in the entire VA system that had reached the pinnacle of NSQIP standings—the coveted "low-outlier status"—in six out of the seven years since implementation of the program had first been reported in medical journals. In Mark's eyes, NSQIP had not only proven that the VA was capable of improvement, it was corroboration of his belief that all measures of VA success would place *his* program at the top of the heap. Little did he suspect that all of that was about to change.

Mark confided a couple of other salient NSQIP-related facts to me over the many years when he considered me a close confidant. First, he let me know that of all VA statistics, NSQIP standing had become the single most important yardstick by which VA hospitals were judged, both regionally and centrally. In other words, the success of any given VA hospital program, and therefore the success of its hospital director and its chief of staff, was judged heavily based on NSQIP standings. There was therefore tremendous pressure on those administrators to do whatever they could to make their hospital's NSQIP results look better—especially as their counterparts at other hospitals were equally desperately doing whatever they could either to catch up or to get further ahead. That pressure, of course, would immediately be transmitted to the chief of the hospital's Surgical Service, sitting one rung down on the local administrative pecking order.

The second, and somewhat related, NSQIP tidbit that Mark imparted to me was that, in addition to the importance of ever-improving NSQIP results for career advancement, annual salary bonuses were also granted to VA hospital chiefs of staffs and to their chiefs of surgical services based on the successes of their hospitals' NSQIP evaluation.

And so, I had gotten some of the clues, an inkling of what the whole NSQIP thing meant to the people who called the shots at the VA, both locally and nationally. But two things stood out in my personal experiences of 2009 and 2010 that made me wonder exactly how important NSQIP statistics really were to the institution: 1) Mark Ratcliffe's increasingly impassioned public and private prohibitions against bringing patients into the operating room for whom the risk of death was more than an extremely remote concern; and 2) the personal warnings I had received against letting even one of my patients die, regardless of the circumstances of the patients' lives and their rights to carefully considered but potentially risky care.

What I was just beginning to understand was that NSQIP was a central part of the VA's mythic story of "transformation." It was therefore a central part of its defense of the institution's status quo before bodies like Congress—and of the justification for its persistent existence in the face of potentially lethal institutional criticism. In other words, NSQIP had become a monolithic entity in the VA program of statistical salvation and self-aggrandizement. It was here to stay.

So what exactly was NSQIP, anyway?

It some ways, it was nothing short of a miracle.

Between the time that the Veterans Administration was formally created by the Hoover administration in 1930 and the time it was converted into a cabinet-level department in 1989, the VA had grown from sixty hospitals to 150. It had become, by far, the biggest healthcare system in the United States, serving millions of members. But there had not been a great deal of planning for that rapid expansion, much of which occurred in the two decades or so after World War II. And unfortunately, the roots of the VA, its history as a safety net for the maimed, homeless, and downtrodden veterans of war, created an indelible impression in the minds of the people who worked at the institution, and of those who collaborated with it: VA patients were essentially second-class citizens whom the nation had deemed worthy of an extra handout. It was not regarded, as it probably should have been, as a national obligation, a debt, to all veterans—and not just to the worst off, an obligation to do everything possible to safeguard the health of the men and women who had defended our country in return for the peril that the nation had inflicted on their physical and mental well-being.

In fact, by the 1980s, the VA had developed a terrible reputation for awful conditions and even for the mistreatment of veterans. Popular films such as *Born on the Fourth of July* depicted horrific conditions at VA hospitals, and although there might have been some dramatic hyperbole, no one really questioned the basic veracity of the observations that people like Oliver Stone were making.

I knew that NSQIP had been born against the backdrop of dissatisfaction with what had become an indefensible VA status quo. But after my personal experiences of 2009 and 2010, I delved deeper into a more detailed understanding of NSQIP, its origins, and what I believed must have been its complex and sophisticated mechanisms of achieving its remarkable success in improving VA surgical outcomes. NSQIP had not simply been initiated by the VA on its own in an attempt to reverse its own downward spiral. Instead, after many decades of decline, conditions at the VA had finally attracted the attention of an irate Congress. In December 1985, a law was enacted demanding that the VA "monitor and evaluate the quality of healthcare furnished by the [VA] Department of Medicine and Surgery." The overarching goal of the new law was to determine whether the quality of VA care deviated, as had been alleged, from "prevailing national standards."[59]

But the "quality of healthcare" was way too enormous and complex a phenomenon to quantitatively measure and compare. Even Congress somehow realized that. Theirs was an unprecedented demand, and there were no existing analytical tools to satisfy it. And so, as its legislative proponents were hashing out this new law, the search must have been on to identify some critical element of patient care that could be quantified and reported back to Congress.

There was nothing easier to diagnose or to demonstrate definitively in medicine than death. But even in evaluating death or survival, there was still a problem: death, in general, is actually a hard medical milestone to improve upon or even to compare because everybody dies. Survival time for many diseases can be very hard to pin down because it's not often clear how long a patient has been suffering with a particular disease before it comes to light. Faced with a conceptual impasse, congressional leaders must have then had an epiphany: surgery.

Every surgery starts at a precise moment on a precise day, a moment that everyone can agree upon. A certain number of patients don't make it through their operations, but even at the VA that number is fairly small. A lot more people will die within a month of an operation, and "thirty-day postoperative mortality" was already a statistic to which surgeons and administrators paid attention. Operations would give the VA a precise moment to start the ticking of a survival clock for each patient who underwent surgery, and the thirty-day point gave them a very reasonable time at which to call each operation either a survival success . . . or a failure.

And so, in an attempt to fulfill its desire for a general assessment of VA care, Congress, in Public Law 99-166, required specifically that the VA determine its own mortality and morbidity rates for all surgical procedures, compare them to "national standards," and then assess whether any deviations from those standards reflected "deficiencies in the quality of healthcare" provided by the VA.[60]

---

[59] Public Law 99-166, Title II, Section 204 (a).

[60] Public Law 99-166, Title II, Section 204 (a).

I found this example of congressional micromanagement to be extraordinary, and a clear reflection of exasperation with what Congress must have been discovering, at least publically, about the reality of a shameful VA. In any event, this was the birth, or at least the moment of conception, of NSQIP.

The great irony of Public Law 99-166, and what no member of the 99th Congress likely realized, was that this well-intentioned congressional demand most likely helped instigate the development within the VA of one of the most powerful weapons in the institution's current arsenal to preserve its status quo. A weapon that not only protects the institution from further criticism and assault, but that often prevents any truly meaningful change or improvement. Public Law 99-166, along with NSQIP and numerous other statistical programs aimed at demonstrations of VA "quality improvement," provided a platform upon which VA leaders could create the appearance of "improvement," and fostered a new VA "tradition" of focusing immense energy and attention on the collection of a limited number of statistics that:

1) could be used to convince Congress and the American people that everything was now fine at the VA; and that

2) may or may not have reflected any real change whatsoever in the overwhelming VA culture of perpetuated mediocrity, a culture that threatened the well-being and even the safety of America's veterans on a regular basis.

Whether they realized the potential consequences or not, Congress attempted to dictate to the VA that it improve the quality of care for every veteran, but in reality Congress decided that they could only dictate that the VA come back to them with a witch's broomstick of good-looking statistics. And if the VA leadership had no idea how to undo decades of a pervasive institutional attitude that supported laziness, indifference, and mediocrity, they might certainly be able to figure out how to make certain specific numbers look good, or at least "better." Congress, in trying to pin the VA down, unintentionally gave it its most formidable way out; they focused attention on one specific measurement of "quality"—in this case, surgical mortality and morbidity—and gave the VA several years and all the money it needed to figure out *how* to make itself look good.

To be fair, there is no indication that NSQIP, and the National VA Surgical Risk Study that preceded it, was initiated with the intention of deceiving Congress, or anyone else. Far from it —there is every indication that it was designed as a completely honest attempt to accomplish something in medicine that had never been done before. Congress, even in the body of Public Law 99-166, acknowledged that the VA was first going to need to create a novel statistical means of comparing outcomes like surgical deaths in hospitals that had very different patient populations, and therefore in hospitals for which you would expect different death rates even if they provided an identical quality of care. In other words, the absolute surgical death rates would need to be statistically *adjusted* for the level of risk inherent in each hospital's unique patient population. This had been done on a national scale by the Society of Thoracic Surgeons for cardiac surgery alone, but nothing so comprehensive had ever been achieved for something as large and complex as all of surgery. And so the first order of business for the VA was the establishment of a method for comprehensive analysis of the practice of surgery in a very large healthcare system, and of a statistically valid method, a so-called "risk adjusted" method, for comparing each hospital's performance within that system.

In order to adjust the statistics based on inherent risk, the VA would need to know a lot about each patient undergoing surgery. And with Congress's blessing and financial support, they did just that. The subsequent collection of more than one hundred important variables on each patient undergoing surgery in such a large system was unprecedented. The statistical analysis of those variables in an attempt to understand which were the most important preoperative characteristics to determine each patient's risk of death or other complication was a milestone of which the VA should have deservedly been proud.

With this enormous statistical machine in place, the VA could now compare the "risk-adjusted" performance of hospitals throughout the system. That meant that at the end of each year, NSQIP could assess almost the entire surgical population at a given hospital and determine how many deaths would have occurred had the hospital been performing exactly at the average of the entire VA system. That calculation was referred to as the "expected" number of deaths. By then counting the actual deaths that had occurred, or that had been "observed," at that same hospital during that year, NSQIP could calculate an "observed-to-expected ratio." An O:E ratio of one meant that the hospital was performing exactly at the average level of the entire VA. If a hospital's O:E ratio was statistically significantly lower than one, it was considered a "low outlier." Low outlier status meant that a hospital had among the very best results of any in the entire VA, and it became a highly sought-after NSQIP distinction. "High outlier" status, on the other hand, with an O:E ratio statistically significantly higher than one, was a sign that something at a hospital was very wrong.

The true accomplishment of NSQIP was the development of a means of predicting the risk of complications in a given hospital's patient population, compared to other hospitals within a closed system. But one irony of NSQIP that I realized only in light of my study of the legislation from which it was derived was that it never actually came close to achieving the one goal that Congress had actually assigned: the comparison of VA care to "prevailing national standards." The impossible problem to solve was simply that no matter how hard the VA worked to analyze its own performance, there was still no national yardstick of surgical outcomes that could serve as a "prevailing national standard" to which the VA outcomes could be compared.

The leadership of the VA and of NSQIP was faced with an impossible task, but rather than throw up their hands and surrender the VA to Congress, they decided to begin with the small initial steps that they could take. There was no national yardstick of surgical outcomes that served as a "prevailing national standard." But the VA could measure everything they could think of about surgery *within the VA system*. Then they could create the unprecedented tool of a "risk adjusted" analysis of all of that VA surgery. The inescapable limitation was that this tool, despite the impressive size of the database from which it was derived, would only be applicable to the system for which it was derived. It would not necessarily tell you anything about the risk of death or complications outside the VA. I surmised in 2010 that if that part of the congressional demand was impossible to satisfy, the VA leadership must have taken the only rational step they could: they ignored it, and hoped everyone else would ignore it, too.

It is not completely clear when the VA leadership realized that with a risk-adjusted model they could compare the performance of different VA hospitals within the VA system. It might truly have been a conscious goal from the beginning. And it was probably true that they hoped to find a way of using information from the "best" VA hospitals to help the "worst" VA hospitals try to do better. Although still not satisfying Congress's demand to know if the VA, *as a whole*, was performing below national standards, this approach of making the worst VA offenders perform a little better promised at least to raise the *average* VA performance, and might have had a chance to appease an otherwise impatient Congress. Of course, if performance everywhere in the VA was below the national standard, all of that effort would fall short of satisfying Congress's true desire to see the veterans' care at least equal that of the rest of the country. But it was all the VA could do, and so they must have hoped that Congress would be satisfied.

Even if the VA leadership of the late 1980s and early 1990s did hope to improve VA performance by identifying the best and worst surgical hospitals, there was still a major problem. Yes, there were known statistical methods for developing a so-called "risk adjusted model" that could potentially be used to compare VA hospitals. But there were no proven, comprehensive, or reliable methods to take the simple ranking of hospitals that would result and use that ranking to improve a complex process like the delivery of surgical care—even just among the worst performers. In the early days, the NSQIP leadership wrote about "guidelines to help the providers [at poor-performing hospitals] conduct structured internal reviews to identify problems in the quality of their surgical care."[61] They encouraged good-performing hospitals to "share with the NSQIP the processes and structures that these hospitals consider to have contributed to their good performance." And in more recent years, they described implementing "observational studies, structured site visits, and follow-ups with feedback to struggling facilities"[62] to try to help those struggling facilities do better. But there has been

---

[61] Khuri SF, Daley J, Hendersoni W, et al. The Department of Veterans Affairs NSQIP. Ann Surg 1998; 228:491-504.

[62] Itani KMF. Fifteen years of the National Surgical Quality Improvement Program in review. Am J. Surg. 2009; 198:S9-18.

little or no documentation over the years of specific things that had been learned or specific steps that had been taken in poor-performing hospitals that had clearly made them better. Instead, what the leaders of NSQIP stumbled upon must have made all of that very difficult stuff suddenly completely irrelevant.

What they stumbled upon was the true miracle of NSQIP. It was certainly too good to be true.

The people at NSQIP began to notice a very interesting pattern: without any sort of concerted, systematic intervention—essentially by telling the good places that they were good and telling the bad places that they were bad—everybody's performance started getting better, and surgical mortality and morbidity was suddenly dropping everywhere across the VA.

Everywhere.

This result exceeded everyone's expectations. Within three years, mortality across the board was down 10 percent, and surgical morbidity had been slashed by about one-third. Again, that was not what Congress had demanded; they wanted parity with "national standards." But those "standards" had never been measured quantitatively, nor was there any means to measure them. And so in lieu of documenting parity, Congress did seem satisfied that the VA had made a very good faith effort to document its own outcomes, and to implement a system that was making things better.

And if those initial 10 percent and 30 percent improvements in mortality and morbidity, respectively, had seemed good, over the course of the next decade, NSQIP reduced VA surgical mortality by 47 percent, and surgical morbidity by 43 percent, without actually doing anything except looking at the data and telling hospitals how they ranked, one against the other.

The real, unspoken question, of course, was whether things were truly, somewhat inexplicably, getting better. And if so, why?

Of course, the VA leadership could not possibly question that the dropping mortality and morbidity numbers were reflective of real improvement across the VA, and a direct result of all the hard work and tax dollars they had poured into NSQIP. After all, not only were careers being made (and saved), but suddenly top VA administrators, rather than hanging their heads low, had something to brag about. Very few systems had ever been able to document this kind of dramatic improvement, particularly one associated with an organized quality improvement program and with such rigorous and complete data. In fact, it was unprecedented. In the absence of a clear, systematic mechanism for this improvement, it was certainly hard to understand. But most top VA administrators, and probably most congresspeople, seemed happy to stick with the bottom line: explanation or no explanation, the numbers were getting better.

But if NSQIP *had* succeeded in lowering surgical morbidity and mortality throughout the VA by simply measuring each hospital's results, there must have been an explanation. In 2010, I began to wonder what that explanation was.

The original idea of bringing concrete, actionable ideas from the "best" places to the "worst" had never really materialized on any meaningful level, so that explanation was out. Besides, that mechanism of improvement would have only explained improvement at the worst hospitals, but that is not what was observed, or heralded. Morbidity and mortality dropped *everywhere*. Instead, the only "official" interpretation of the NSQIP phenomenon has been that people do a better job if you tell them that they're being watched, or perhaps if you focus their own attention on what they are doing.

Really?

As I explored what has been written about NSQIP, I found references to the "Hawthorne Effect." As I read more about the Hawthorne Effect, I thought about Shukri Khuri, the VA elder statesman who was the leader of, and who became considered the mastermind of, NSQIP, and with whom I'd had the chance to work at the West Roxbury VA during my general surgery residency at Harvard. I could just imagine a look of great relief spreading across Shukri's face as one of his colleagues, or perhaps even a research assistant, came running into his office one day, shouting, "I've got it, I've got—the explanation for all the improvement we're seeing in NSQIP! It's called the 'Hawthorne Effect!'"

So what was the Hawthorne Effect? It turned out to be a relatively obscure, and controversial, if not actually discredited, psychological phenomenon that had been observed in experimental industrial settings in the 1920s and early '30s. Workers who were part of experimental programs designed to assess the relationship between productivity and various working conditions became more productive whenever the conditions were changed. The improvements tended to be short lived, but the real indictment of the data came when the researchers changed conditions back to the original state, and productivity improved again! Since the conditions themselves could not therefore explain the improvement, it was hypothesized that the workers reacted transiently with a more productive effort simply in response to the perception of being observed.

Shukri Khuri probably did not care very much that the validity of the Hawthorne Effect has remained on the controversial fringe of mainstream psychology. Here it was, a published psychological phenomenon that might explain the otherwise inexplicable improvement in VA surgical numbers. But, I wondered, even if factory workers do work harder for a brief period of time when they are first told that they are being watched, could that phenomenon truly provide an explanation for an ongoing, dramatic improvement in such an extremely complex and multifactorial process as the delivery of surgical care? A process that involved the interplay of so many disparate groups of professionals? To me, it just didn't seem plausible. But any other explanation involving the mere identification of sub-par performers failed to account for the reduction in mortality and morbidity that was seen across the board, even at programs that were not being flagged for poor performance at all.

Any other explanation, that was, except for one.

I began to wonder if people truly had an untapped, almost limitless capacity for coordinated self-improvement, so that all you had to do is tell them that someone was watching. I wondered if such a capacity could possibly emerge spontaneously across an entire, complex organization, an organization as big and as complicated as the surgical operation of a VA hospital?

Or did people who were already used to checking boxes as a means of documenting the value of their work, people who were already satisfied with making their work *look* satisfactory even if they knew that things were done better elsewhere, instead have an untapped capacity to find ways of making things look even better when they were told exactly what was being watched—and how.

Suddenly I thought about the innumerable times I had sat through Mark Ratcliffe's public and private exhortations for his staff to refrain from bringing any patient to the operating room if there was a perceived chance that the patient might die. Until 2010, I hadn't fully realized how critical NSQIP had been in saving the VA from an unprecedented threat of congressional impatience and dissatisfaction, and therefore how central the program had become to the VA leadership's perception of institutional survival. I had never thought about how effectively that central VA leadership had transmitted the importance of this program to the attitudes and actions of local administrators on the front lines of data collection, and data *generation*. Simply put, I had never realized how much attention was focused on that specific aspect of each VA hospital's performance.

Suddenly, NSQIP seemed less like a VA administrative curiosity, and instead like something potentially more sinister.

Finally, after decades of unquestioned, complacent mediocrity, the VA had faced a congressional demand for scrutiny. Surgical leaders throughout the VA knew that a harsh spotlight had been turned on. They also knew what was being measured, and they knew what their bosses wanted to see. The only way to avoid surgical mortality altogether was not to operate at all. Short of that, the second best way to reduce mortality was to refuse surgery to the patients who were more likely to die, whether or not they were the most deserving or in the most desperate need of surgery. Whether or not the VA had explicitly been given the responsibility for carrying out the inevitably higher risk care of veterans who inherently made up a high-risk population. Whether or not the nation had made one promise to all veterans: to provide the healthcare that they needed and wanted, regardless of any other adverse conditions in their lives.

What was most fascinating to me was the way Mark had told the members of the Surgical Service that the prohibition against high-risk surgery was not his idea, nor was our compliance a matter of choice. The VA had decided, he would tell us, that we were not to engage in very high-risk cases, and since we were employees of the VA, Mark firmly believed that we had no choice but to comply with VA "policy." Whatever we chose to do in our roles as independent practitioners outside of the VA, once inside his hospital's four walls, we needed to do as we were told. I was sure that there had never been a memo circulated to Mark or any other chiefs of VA surgical services indicating a "policy" of avoiding high-risk surgery. Instead, Mark was reacting to all of the attention that must have been focused in his own administrative meetings with people like Diana Nicoll, in which an ongoing improvement in NSQIP statistics must have been delineated clearly as one of the hospital's single most important priorities. One thing was clear to Mark: both Diana Nicoll and her own superiors in the VA hierarchy wanted to see fewer surgical deaths. Period.

The greatest accomplishment of NSQIP, again ironically, had not been a leveling of the VA playing field, in which poor performers learned how to be more like the best. That was what the NSQIP leaders had hypothesized might be possible, that was the only thing that might have made sense. But a separation between poor performers and good performers persisted. Instead, the great accomplishment of NSQIP was the reduction of raw, "unadjusted" mortality and morbidity rates throughout the VA. But if some of that miracle had been achieved through the avoidance of risky surgeries, wouldn't NSQIP's elaborate system of measuring risk factors have picked up a drop in those risks?

And more to the point, if individual hospitals were judged and compared not based on raw, "unadjusted" mortality, but on the "O:E" ratio of observed deaths to expected deaths, wouldn't the avoidance of risky cases fail to game the system, since lower risk cases would drop not only the number of observed deaths, but also the number of expected deaths, as well?

By the same token, wouldn't it be okay for a hospital to lose high-risk patients, since the performance of their surgeries allowed the hospital's number of expected deaths to rise?

The answer to all these questions is related to the statistical problem of small numbers. Risk adjustment most effectively ameliorates the impact of high-risk deaths when one considers a large system like the entire VA, where there might be more than one hundred thousand surgeries in a single year and therefore more than one thousand deaths. But when considering just one hospital performing less than one thousand cases—a hospital that is expected to match a national average of less than 1.5 percent overall mortality—the implication is that there have got to be fewer than fifteen operative deaths. Suddenly, every single death becomes very important to the calculation, because one simply does not have the large denominator of other cases to balance things out statistically. Over many years, the impact of the high-risk cases on the hospital's calculation of expected deaths might help, but there is no guarantee in any given year that several high-risk deaths wouldn't push the O:E ratio right out of the highly coveted, "low-outlier" territory.

The safest thing for any hospital to do was simply to avoid as many deaths as possible, and therefore to avoid the patients at higher risk. And as years went by and *everybody's* numbers kept getting miraculously better, the pressure would rise more and more to make sure that only the least risky cases were actually getting done.

Faced with an imperative to keep up with systemwide improvements in NSQIP statistics, there was something else that hospitals could do. The relative importance of different NSQIP risk factors was published every year, and even though in theory that relative importance could change from year to year, it rarely did. And so hospital administrators and surgeons knew what factors would make their patients look like they were higher or lower risk. There has never been any evidence that local VA administrators ever instructed their dedicated NSQIP nurses to alter any of the data they collected. In fact, independent audits have verified that NSQIP data very closely match the data in the patients' medical records. But it turned out that four out of the five risk factors that contributed the most to each patient's calculation of risk, year in and year out, were factors that were judged and assigned subjectively by the VA doctors that were performing the surgeries or administering anesthesia. Things like the patient's class of anesthesia risk, which the anesthesiologist alone determined based mostly on his or her personal judgment. Things like whether the operation was considered an "emergency" or not. Things like the "complexity score" of the operation, and the "functional status" of the patient. Those surgeons and anesthesiologists knew that their own work would be judged more critically if they routinely assigned subjective numbers to their patients that made them look "lower risk." The assignment of these numbers was very subjective to begin with. Even without a conscious desire to influence the NSQIP analysis, practitioners might very well subconsciously want to get credit for what they already perceived as "high-risk" work. Without realizing it, people might even have become less aggressive about describing certain nonlethal complications in their official hospital notes.

What I began to realize as I learned more and more about the guts of NSQIP was that it was perfectly suited for a VA in which appearances were everything, and at which there were no inherent expectations for outstanding performance. I realized that "gaming" the system would not even require any sort of elaborate, national conspiracy, but that it was the likely, if not inevitable outcome, of the VA system just doing what it did best. Was it truly clear, as NSQIP leaders claimed, that telling hospitals that they were doing a good job or a lousy job actually made everybody somehow perform better? Not at all. Were there more reasonable explanations for why the numbers kept getting better and better, even if VA attitudes and performance had remained largely the same? Certainly there were.

And ironically, the early academic papers that leaders at the VA published in medical journals about NSQIP and its remarkable success acknowledged the possibility that there could be gaming of the system, that risk factors might be fudged, and that risky cases might be increasingly avoided. Although they attempted to downplay the possibility, it was impossible to prove that these phenomena were not taking place. That uncertainty, in fact, may have kept the NSQIP publications out of the top mainstream medical journals, such as the *New England Journal of Medicine*—despite their remarkable results—and relegated the papers to publication in less highly regarded "surgical journals." Regardless, I found it curious that even surgical leaders, and much less Congress, had seemed perfectly happy to accept the miracle of the Hawthorne Effect without more vociferously considering much simpler, more obvious, and much more disturbing explanations for the "remarkable" results.

What about the patients? Were their interests, in fact, well served if the VA had limited surgical deaths by avoiding high-risk surgeries? Maybe, if the patients were not able to understand the risks they were facing going into surgery, and if they would have chosen to forgo the operation in order to avoid the chance of not making it through. But that is why the concept of informed consent had become a central tenet of modern medicine. Patients undergo surgeries for very specific reasons, reasons that are at least good enough to justify inevitable pain and suffering. It is the obligation of all surgeons to explain the risks to their patients in great enough detail so that the patients are able to judge the risks and decide if the potential benefits of a painful operation outweigh all of the risks, including death. In our society, the patient is given the right to choose to accept risks in order to gain the corresponding benefits, at least outside the VA.

In 2010, I began to wonder why the VA leadership, Congress, and even the academic community of medical experts who had touched the heralding of this great accomplishment in some direct or indirect way hadn't been asking much tougher questions. If the incredible VA interpretation of NSQIP was wrong, and if, in fact, surgical statistics had been improved primarily through denial of surgical care to those who needed it the most, or, worse yet, through the intentional or even unintentional manipulation of data, then not only was this a crime against scientific integrity, but it was yet another example of the abuse of America's veterans for whom the VA was being asked to answer in the first place.

* * *

With increasingly disturbing questions in my mind about the true impact of NSQIP, I began to wonder more about other aspects of the VA "transformation" that, like NSQIP, had been lauded as a tremendous victory for the VA in response to the congressional dissatisfaction of the 1980s. A transformation that *had*, in fact, been published in the *New England Journal*.

One of the things about the VA "transformation" that seemed most incongruous to me at first blush were the yearly reports of VA patient satisfaction statistics that were the highest in the United States. Reports of statistics that were gathered not by the VA, but by truly objective third-party observers. Although things had gotten better compared to Oliver Stone's horrific depiction of a VA of the 1970s, it was obvious to just about anyone who worked in the VA that the services provided to veterans fell short of the care experienced by patients at the university hospital, or other venues in the private sector.

An explanation for this conundrum hit me one day when I realized that the source for all of the patient satisfaction data were survey answers from the patients themselves. Then I thought about an analogy from a common circumstance of customer dissatisfaction, the check-in counter at San Francisco International Airport.

I imagined the long lines at SFO during a busy time for the airlines. On the one side I imagined a family of four, with a little boy and a girl, whose clothes, baggage, and demeanor all indicated that they did not hail from the swanky part of town. In fact, one could tell that this family probably didn't do too much flying. I assumed, in fact, that the father of this family had done some sort of big favor for his boss at work, and that his boss was so grateful that he bought their whole family tickets to visit Grandma and Grandpa, using just a small fraction of his unused frequent flyer miles.

I imagined this family in line, with the kids getting bored and starting to drive Mom and Dad crazy. The luggage was pretty heavy, and when they finally got to the front of the line, the airline attendant had trouble finding their reservation. Then it was realized that their flight had been cancelled, but the attendant told them that the airline would do what it could. If they waited at the gate for just a few hours, they'd be pushed closer to the top of a standby list for a similar flight.

Then I imagined that on the other side, the part of the counter where first-class passengers and platinum-plus frequent flyers check in, there was a couple in their fifties wearing nothing but Burberry, Hermes, and Prada. This couple had breezed through a nonexistent line and had their bags picked up for them by an obsequious skycap. Now when the airline attendant, addressing them respectfully by their names, checked them in for the same flight, she, too, discovered that the flight had been cancelled. This time, however, she let them know that they had already been rebooked on another flight that would leave just an hour later and that they were welcome to wait in the first-class lounge.

I asked myself which of these two groups of travelers would be more appreciative of the service that they'd received, and which would be cursing the airline under their breath as they strolled toward the TSA checkpoint? The answer seemed obvious. The family that usually subsided on very little would still be excited about visiting Grandma and Grandpa for free, and even though they were a little screwed and were going to have to put up with a lot more hardship, they would still be pretty happy about what they got.

But the snooty rich people who always expect to be treated well and who paid through the nose for an overpriced first-class ticket would not be too likely to appreciate the way that people bent over backwards to make them comfortable. Instead they would be more likely to be irked that the airline had once again, albeit ever so slightly, messed up their plans.

And so, if someone shoved a customer satisfaction survey in front of both of those imaginary parties, it was quite clear to me that the family that had suffered through a tougher experience would still give the airline a higher score than the couple who had been handled like royalty.

It was not necessarily the care at the VA that was responsible for its high patient satisfaction data; it could very well have been the veterans themselves. I had learned many times that veterans, as a group, were used to getting the short end of the stick, and they were used to receiving little or nothing in return for their own sacrifices and hard work. So when they finally did get something of value, and especially when they believed that they were getting something for free that other people had to pay for (or at least at a substantially reduced cost), there was no question in my mind that they would be more likely to be "satisfied." In general, the veterans were an incredibly appreciative bunch. It was clear that they would be much more likely to appreciate the care they received at the VA than many patients who came to our university clinics with high expectations, and who were often put off by a long wait or a less than perfectly attentive doctor or nurse. The vets did tend to appreciate everything, and no matter how poor the service might have been, they'd often tell you it was better than a kick in the teeth.

What struck me as particularly brilliant of the VA was the manner in which it played up and publicized its patient satisfaction results without ever drawing attention to this simple and undeniable observation.

But if the vets were a large part of the explanation for the VA's highly touted patient satisfaction success, there was still an element of the "transformation" that needed explaining. Despite the fact that my own observations of care at the VA hadn't changed at all significantly in the twenty years I had been exposed to the institution, the VA was also being hailed for among the highest scores in the country on third-party measurements of quality of care. These data, of course, were more "objective" and did not originate from the patients.

This time, the explanation came not from the source of data, but from the methods by which such a measurement was being attempted in the first place. Congress had found it unreasonable even to ask the VA to measure the quality of its overall care, and instead had demanded data only on the VA's thirty-day surgical morbidity and mortality. If even such a small, single aspect of care proved so difficult and so expensively cumbersome to measure, how could anyone possibly attempt to measure something as enormous and vague as the quality of medical care in general?

One might attempt to measure quality of care based entirely on outcomes, perhaps on how many people live or die, or how many get bad complications of their diseases. But the risk adjustment that was necessary for the VA to look at surgical outcomes would be impossibly prohibitive to attempt for all of medicine. Without risk adjustment, the comparison of results from different patient populations would not be meaningful.

Since outcomes were not available as a means to measure the quality of care for all of medicine, the academic and practical analysis of quality of care has had to focus instead on certain specific details of care that can be systematically observed and measured. The hope is that those small details would reflect back on the totality of care that is provided in any given system as a whole.

For example, to measure the quality of inpatient care, one cannot look at all of the hundreds of diagnoses that bring people into the hospital. Instead, a few types of medical problems are selected, such as heart attacks or pneumonia, and attention is focused on those few. The assumption is that hospitals that do a good job at taking care of heart attacks probably do a good job at taking care of urinary tract infections and gallstones, too. Even with heart attacks it is impossible for an observer to assess everything about the patients' care, and so, again, certain details of the care are selected for observation, such as how soon the patients are given aspirin after a heart attack and how many of the patients leave the hospital having been prescribed certain benchmark drugs. Once again, the assumption is that a good job on these details reflects a decent job on everything else involved in taking care of a heart attack victim.

The ideal design of this type of system of very selective quality surveillance would not allow the doctors under observation to know which specific details of which specific diseases were being measured. In fact, it would be best to keep the doctors and the hospitals in the dark, and keep them guessing what might be measured next. That way, they'd have to do everything as well as possible, since they wouldn't know which small aspect of their care would be scrutinized. Ideally, the focuses of observation would be changed often and without notice, in order to get the clearest picture of what was really going on.

The reality is, however, that everyone at the VA knows which diseases are being monitored, and everyone knows which details are being observed. In fact, numerous hospital employees receive salary bonuses when specific indices of quality of care reach certain specified benchmarks. Nurses have been assigned to monitor just those specific details of care and provide real-time feedback to clinical teams to make sure that things looked as good as possible at the moment when success or failure for a given patient was being recorded. Thus, the explanation for the inordinate amount of attention paid to each bypass patient's blood sugar level at six a.m. on the morning after surgery. And the explanation for the complete lack of attention paid to the innumerable elements of care that were not being monitored or recorded, such as how quickly patients could get tests or referred for consults before an operation could be scheduled. Or how much attention was paid by the nurses working the nighttime shifts.

Of course, by allowing the institution to focus attention and energy just on the details it knew were being monitored, the resulting data didn't actually reflect at all on the vast majority of the institution's care, and the value of the entire endeavor was lost. Outstanding six a.m. blood sugar levels told us nothing about the true quality of VA care, even about the care of post-bypass patients. Even worse, the rest of the care in the hospital might very well have gotten worse and worse, as more and more resources were focused on the few details being monitored, and attention and resources were inevitably drawn away from the multitude of important details that didn't have any influence on anyone's annual bonus.

But the particularly ironic aspect of this ineffective method of trying to gauge the overall quality of care was that the VA's "success" at mastering this obvious gaming created an illusion of quality that staved off Congress's very justified dissatisfaction and demands for real improvement. Instead of improving the system, the entire process likely reduced or eliminated any chance of the meaningful, sweeping, and pervasive changes that are truly needed — and that our veterans truly deserve.

ACKNOWLEDGMENTS

No one involved in the creation of this book deserves more thanks or more credit than my family, and especially my wife, Rui Meng, who instilled in me the courage to stand up for what is right, and then the strength and determination not to give up. Right behind her have been my parents, Abraham and Florence Mann, who were subjected to endless drafts and even more endless brainstorming sessions. I must thank Ave Butensky, whose unbridled, unflinching support for the project and whose remarkable network both proved indispensable in getting from concept to finished book. Along the way, I had the incredibly good fortune to learn an entirely new craft from editor, collaborator and friend Tony Koltz, and was equally lucky to receive the support, inspiration and guidance of Mel Berger at William Morris Endeavor. I am also grateful to Dr. Fred Frank for his availability, his affability and his advice, to Hilary Claggett, and to the folks at Mill City Press for their contributions to the book's eventual publication.

Of course, there are many people who deserve my deepest gratitude for their support of my cause, not the least of whom are Drs. Nancy Ascher and David Jablons at UCSF, my stalwart attorneys and advisers Kurt Melchior and Gregg Cochran, and my dear friends Joel and Paula Blank. But as a citizen of the United States, I will always remain most grateful to the men and women who have served in our armed forces, for the sacrifices they make on our behalf, and on behalf of a safer, more secure world.